R0006170252

| Wallace Library | DUE DATE (stamped in blue) |
	RETURN DATE (stamped in black)
MAY 24 1997	
APR 2 4 1998	
OCT 3 1 1998	
NOV 0 2 1998	
APR 2 4 2000 APR 2 8 2000	
FEB 2 6 2001	
FEB 1 2 2001	
JAN 0 3 2005	

D1468378

Computers in Health Care

Kathryn J. Hannah   Marion J. Ball
Series Editors

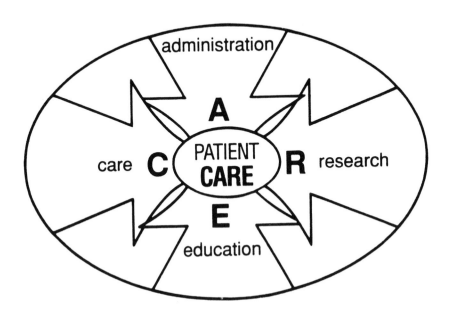

Computers in Health Care

Series Editors:
Kathryn J. Hannah   Marion J. Ball

Nursing Informatics
Where Caring and Technology Meet
M.J. Ball, K.J. Hannah, U. Gerdin Jelger, and H. Peterson

Healthcare Information Management Systems
A Practical Guide
M.J. Ball, J.V. Douglas, R.I. O'Desky, and J.W. Albright

Knowledge Coupling
New Premises and New Tools for Medical Care and Education
Lawrence L. Weed

Dental Informatics
Integrating Technology into the Dental Environment
Louis M. Abbey and John Zimmerman

Aspects of the Computer-based Patient Record
Marion J. Ball and Morris F. Collen

Introduction to Nursing Informatics
K.J. Hannah, M.J. Ball, and M.J.A. Edwards

Strategy and Architecture of Health Care Information Systems
Michael K. Bourke

Organizational Aspects of Health Informatics
Managing Technological Change
Nancy M. Lorenzi and Robert T. Riley

Patient Care Information Systems
Successful Design and Implementation
Erica L. Drazen, Jane B. Metzer, Jami
L. Ritter, and Mark K. Schneider

Nancy M. Lorenzi
Robert T. Riley

Organizational Aspects of Health Informatics

Managing Technological Change

With 25 illustrations

Springer-Verlag

New York Berlin Heidelberg London Paris
Tokyo Hong Kong Barcelona Budapest

Nancy M. Lorenzi
Associate Senior Vice President
University of Cincinnati
  Medical Center
231 Bethesda Avenue
Cincinnati, OH 45267 USA

Robert T. Riley
President, Riley Associates
221 Hilltop Lane
Cincinnati, OH 45215
USA

Library of Congress Cataloging-in-Publication Data
Lorenzi, Nancy M.
        Organizational aspects of health informatics : managing
    technological change / Nancy M. Lorenzi, Robert T. Riley.
            p. cm. - (Computers in health care)
        Includes bibliographical references and index.
        ISBN 0-387-94226-2. -- ISBN 3-540-94226-2
        1. Medical informatics. 2. Health services administration.
    I. Riley, Robert T., II. Title. III. Series: Computers in health
    care (New York, N.Y.)
    R858.L67 1994   94-19977
    362.1'0285--dc20

Printed on acid-free paper.

© 1995 Springer-Verlag New York, Inc.
All rights reserved. This work may not be translated or copied in whole or in part without the written permission of the publisher (Springer-Verlag New York, Inc., 175 Fifth Avenue, New York, NY
10010, USA), except for brief excerpts in connection with reviews or scholarly analysis. Use in connection with any form of information storage and retrieval, electronic adaptation, computer software, or by similar or dissimilar methodology now known or hereafter developed is forbidden.
The use of general descriptive names, trade names, trademarks, etc., in this publication, even if the
former are not especially identified, is not to be taken as a sign that such names, as understood by
the Trade Marks and Merchandise Marks Act, may accordingly be used freely by anyone.

Production managed by Karen Phillips; manufacturing supervised by Gail Simon.
Camera-ready copy provided by the authors.
Printed by Edwards Brothers, Inc., Ann Arbor, MI.
Printed in the United States of America.

9 8 7 6 5 4 3 2 1

ISBN 0-387-94226-2 Springer-Verlag New York Berlin Heidelberg
ISBN 3-540-94226-2 Springer-Verlag Berlin Heidelberg New York

*To all those who have learned the hard way
that hardware and software are not enough*

Series Preface

This series is intended for the rapidly increasing number of health care professionals who have rudimentary knowledge and experience in health care computing and are seeking opportunities to expand their horizons. It does not attempt to compete with the primers already on the market. Eminent international experts will edit, author or contribute to each volume in order to provide comprehensive and current accounts of innovations and future trends in this quickly evolving field. Each book will be practical, easy to use, and well referenced.

Our aim is for the series to encompass all of the health professions by focusing on specific professions, such as nursing, in individual volumes. However, integrated computing systems are only one tool for improving communication among members of the health care team. Therefore, it is our hope that the series will stimulate professionals to explore additional means of fostering interdisciplinary exchange.

This series springs from a professional collaboration that has grown over the years into a highly valued personal friendship. Our joint values put people first. If the Computers in Health Care series lets us share those values by helping health care professionals to communicate their ideas for the benefit of patients, then our efforts will have succeeded.

Kathryn J. Hannah
Marion J. Ball

Acknowledgments

As we were writing this book, we thought several times about the need to acknowledge the assistance we have received from so many people. When the "gallows humor" effect inevitably took over at times during the process, we laughed about the types of comments we might make, ranging from thanking every relative whose name we could remember to thanking those—especially, the guilty—who figured in many of the "war stories" scattered throughout the book.

However, as our writing process on this book draws to a close, we appreciate our debts to all those who have supported our writing effort. We hope that this book will aid in creating more successful health informatics implementations over the coming decade, and we also hope that we can help reduce the "pains" and "scars" that we and others have suffered in the past in this area. Thus, our acknowledgments are truly from the heart.

Our first acknowledgment must be to Dr. Marion J. Ball, President of IMIA and co-editor of this Springer-Verlag series with Dr. Kathryn J. Hannah. Marion has an uncanny sense of timing as to when issues are right for further exploration and when people need to be nurtured and encouraged into making a contribution. Our relationship with Marion began in the 1970s when she and Nancy served on the National Library of Medicine's Biomedical Library Review Committee. For many years, the relationship continued only through an annual Christmas message. However, when most needed, Marion became reconnected more intensely with our lives, and there have been many positive outcomes of this reconnection. This book is only one. To Marion, our heartfelt thanks and love.

Another critical supporter has been Dr. Donald C. Harrison, Senior Vice President and Provost of the University of Cincinnati Medical Center. Don has not only supported Nancy's expansion into new areas and responsibilities, but he also supported a yearlong sabbatical so that she could focus on organizing an International Working Conference on the Organizational Impact of Informatics as well as beginning the writing of this book. Without that sabbatical, neither would have been possible. Don participated in the Working Conference and is currently utilizing Nancy's change management and organizational development expertise in a wide range of areas at the Medical Center.

We must also thank the participants at the 1993 International Medical Informatics Association Working Conference on the Organizational Impact of Informatics. This Working Conference clarified for us that there is a real need for a book in this area and provided a wealth of materials. Some of the participants came because they had a long commitment to the people side of technology; some came because of the enthusiastic evangelizing of two members of the conference planning committee, Dr. Peter N. Rosen of Kaiser Permanente and Mr. Victor Peel of the University of Manchester; some came as an act of faith in the conference organizers; and some probably came out of pure curiosity. Whatever their reasons, it was an important experience for us, and we thank everyone who participated.

We would especially like to acknowledge Dr. Alan F. Dowling, of Ernst and Young, whose personal, professional, and financial support added to the success of the conference and to some of the directions within this book; Mr. Brad Dixon (soon to be Dr. Brad we hope), from the University of Western Ontario, who has an encyclopedic knowledge of the literature and theoretical concepts in this area; Dr. Bernard Horak, of Horak Associates and George Washington University, who came as a substitute speaker and ended up making a major contribution and becoming a friend; and Dr. Thomas S. Fischer, of Kaiser Permanente, who contributed significantly to the program both intellectually and financially.

Although both of us have written extensively in the past, this is our first book. Without the support and good humored "nagging" by Ms. Andrea Seils, our Springer-Verlag editor, we may well not have persevered through the project. On the technical side, we thank Ms. Karen Phillips and Mr. Ken Dreyhaupt for all their assistance—and flexibility.

We must also formally acknowledge each other. We found that after many years of marriage, we still work together very well on large professional projects. It is a good feeling.

Finally, we do need to grudgingly recognize the "assistance" of all those organizational problem children we have encountered who must remain anonymous—though the temptation is almost overwhelming at times to name names. It is their behaviors and attitudes that either cause or aggravate many of the problems discussed in this book. So to all those people that have provided some of our greatest frustrations over the years—thank you. Without your behaviors, our efforts may never have become so focused.

Contents

Series Preface   vii
Acknowledgments   ix

Section I   Health Care, Organizations, and Informatics   1

1   What's the Problem?   3
2   Stress and Change Management in Implementing
    Health Informatics   19
3   Today's Health Care Environment   35

Section II   Organizational Issues   51

4   Operating in Different Organizational Structures   53
5   Preparing the Organization for Change   75
6   Determining the Strategic Direction   103
7   Some Critical Issues in Project Planning and
    Management   117
8   Change Management for Successful Implementation   149
9   Negotiating the Political Minefields   162

Section III   People Issues   183

10   The Critical Role of Leaders and Leadership   185
11   Preparing the Staff for New Technologies   208
12   Building Effective Teams of Health Professionals   223
13   Managing Personal Stress   235

Section IV   Managing the Project End Stages   253

14   Dealing with End Stage People Issues   255
15   Evaluating Project Success   267
16   Managing the Altered Organization   277

Section V   Future Issues   293

17   Organizational and Personal Preparation
     for the Future   295

Index   306

Section I
Health Care, Organizations, and Informatics

Introduction

Chapter 1 is an overview of the basic problem—too many health informatics implementations are less than completely successful —and its causes.

Chapter 2 presents some of the issues of organizational change and resistance to change common to virtually any organization and presents the relationships between organizational stress, organizational change, and informatics implementations.

Chapter 3 presents some of the unique issues encountered within a health care environment. This chapter is particularly valuable for those having information backgrounds but limited knowledge of the health care environment.

1
What's the Problem?

Do any of these stories seem familiar?

Tale #1

A large hospital in the United States hired a new president who had quite limited knowledge of computers. This hospital had previously tried unsuccessfully to implement a hospital information system (HIS). The new president set the HIS area as a top priority and hired a friend and former colleague whom he trusted as his chief information officer (CIO). A flamboyant character to say the least, this new CIO swept into the organization, loudly announcing that he had come to bring enlightenment to the technological barbarians. At the more personal level, he often lamented loudly and long to anyone who would listen about the horrors of living amid provincials, far from his beloved and sophisticated home.

After considerable deliberation, the CIO selected a system from a new division of an established older company that had no experience in the health care industry. Further, the decision was made with little or no user input and with limited inputs from the managers of the other major systems with which the HIS had to connect.

The hospital president strongly supported his CIO's choice, and millions of dollars were spent on the new system. The systems people were never able to get this system to work. One disastrous crash followed another. Finally, the hardware was sold for pennies on the dollar, and the CIO rode off into the sunrise toward his beloved home.

Incidentally, the same hospital then selected another person to head its computer efforts and settled for much more modest goals. Instead of an HIS, the hospital implemented a basic hospital accounting system that satisfied its administrative needs. However, the clinical staff, with hopes raised by previous wild promises, was left unsatisfied and frustrated.

Tale #2

A major academic medical center was faced with selecting and purchasing a powerful mainframe relational database package with a so-called fourth generation language to serve as the institution's database standard for the future. The selection process narrowed to two choices.

The users—many of them fairly sophisticated—favored a package that was already emerging as a leader and semi-standard in the field. Further, it was the one that many medical equipment manufacturers appeared to be moving toward using or at least supporting. Also, there were more people available who were skilled in this system and more training opportunities available for the unskilled.

The information systems (IS) department "techies" instead fell in love with a more complex, more costly system that they declared to be "technically superior." Since they controlled the money for this particular purchase, their selection was the winner. The system was purchased and extensive training was conducted among the techies.

Most of the users then proceeded one by one to go their own ways using their original choice on powerful smaller systems. Only those applications developed by the IS department used the new system.

As an aside, this same IS department had previously selected a rather obscure database program as the organizational standard to support at the microcomputer level rather than either the traditional industry standard or the emerging new standard. Again, the argument was that their choice was technically superior. Users wishing to benefit from public domain applications developed by colleagues at other institutions rebelled and bought "unsupported" database packages, ignoring the IS dictum.

Tale #3

A large Canadian teaching hospital installed a $13.5 million information system called OSCAR (Online System for Communi-cation And Records). This new system required physicians to enter all their orders into the system—a significant change in procedure. Whether real or not, the perceived reason was the reduction of data entry costs.

In the early implementation stages, the system falsely generated orders for blood transfusions; however, these errors were caught by human intervention so no patient harm was done. Still this was a major rallying point for the system opponents. The critics further charged the system with being old technology and therefore cumbersome and time-consuming to operate, thus lengthening the residents' work days. The video screens were poor, the printers were too noisy, the training was inadequate, etc. In addition, the hospital had elected not to include some modules such as special warnings about patients with similar names.

OSCAR's implementation provoked a bitter two-year conflict between the medical staff—especially the residents—and the hospital administration. The residents proudly wore badges bearing a diagonal bar (the international symbol for "No") over the word "OSCAR." Constant negative comparisons were made to the systems in use at another local hospital. The OSCAR implementation had significantly changed the way work was done for a significant hospital constituency, and these people loudly and openly rebelled.[1]

Tale #4

In the United Kingdom, the Wessex region of the National Health Service (NHS) has been charged with wasting up to £63 million in a ten-year program to perform a major upgrade of its information systems. Even the officials of the system concede that £20 million has been wasted. The charges included the following: there were "secret" removals of penalty clauses from contracts, there were major undisclosed conflicts of interest in the process, there were contracts awarded and subsequently withdrawn after high-powered lobbying, and there were privatization plans developed that guaranteed profits based upon inflated costs.

As this scandal has unfolded, accusations and excuses have filled the newspapers. Numerous heads have rolled among both senior staff and appointed board members, and civil suits for over £5 million have been filed against some private contractors.

Unfortunately, this information management disaster has not been an isolated example. During the past two years, the NHS has suffered several other major, widely publicized financial and/or performance scandals as it has attempted to rapidly upgrade its overall information processing systems. The ultimate danger is the public becoming increasingly disillusioned with the ability of NHS to manage itself effectively. In the past several years, the NHS has spent over £500 million in upgrading the information systems in just 260 major hospitals. If more significant scandals erupt around these huge expenditures, the future of the NHS as it currently exists may well be in danger.[2]

What's a "Failure"?

Many of you can probably match or even top these stories. Unfortunately, there is nothing unusual about them. Many of our health care institutions have consumed huge amounts of money and frustrated countless people in wasted information systems efforts.

"Failure" is a very broad term. Many health informatics projects are certainly not *complete* failures. At some point, the new system is finally installed, becomes operational, and continues to work at some level of performance and user satisfaction. However, there are at least two potential problems:

- Is the system as good as it might have been for the resources expended?
- How much did the system really cost when *all* the costs are considered, including intangibles such as stress on the organization and the individuals involved?

For the purposes of this book, we define a *successful* health informatics implementation as one that meets *both* of the following two criteria:

- A successful health informatics systems implementation meets the standard project management criteria, i.e., it is accomplished on time, within budget, and to technical specifications.
- A successful health informatics systems implementation meets the perceived needs of over 90 percent of the end users, viewed randomly. "Randomly" is used here to indicate that any dissatisfaction is scattered and not concentrated in a particular segment of the end-user group.

These are stringent criteria. Historically, few health informatics projects have met them. Still, they establish a goal of excellence against which all of us can measure our outcomes and our progress toward excellence in this area.

Why Do These Failures Happen?

There are no easy answers as to why so many health informatics projects are not more successful. In most cases, there are multiple factors at play. Even with an in-depth analysis, separating the impacts of these various factors may be possible. Not only do two wrongs not make a right, they may create a third wrong far larger than the sum of the original two—a prime example of negative synergy at work. We can classify the failure factors into three broad categories: technical shortcomings, project management short-comings, and organizational issues shortcomings.

Technical Shortcomings

In the 1990s, a serious issue for many health care IS departments is a lack of basic technical competence in modern information technologies. The rate of change in the information systems area is truly astounding. Some of us can even remember functioning in the BC era—Before Computers. It is hard to realize that the first nongovernmental computer in the world was installed only forty years ago, and the capabilities of that machine were ludicrous by today's standards.

Since that time, the only constant has been change. Some information professionals have delighted in that change and the resulting challenges for continued personal growth and learning. Others have not. They have stopped growing at some point on the improvement curve and are attempting to spend their remaining professional years in their personal comfort zones.

The paradoxical aspect of this problem is that those IS departments that were pioneers are often the most prone to subsequent obsolescence. However, the problem of keeping IS technology current is not so simple for institutions that have significant IS histories of more than ten to fifteen years. The issue of *installed base* can become a massive drag against progress. Anyone can sit down for a few minutes with pencil and paper and determine that the percentage of total IS effort that must go into maintaining previously developed software expands incredibly rapidly as a few years pass. The more difficult that old software is to maintain, the worse the problem. Many IS shops have significant numbers of people using out-of-date COBOL skills to maintain large amounts of out-of-date COBOL software.

When a traditional IS organization attempts to upgrade its software approach, it encounters several problems. It has a massive base of existing software—often referred to as its *legacy* systems—that it cannot just abandon overnight. Until the new software is developed or purchased, the old software must be maintained. The next problem is upgrading the existing staff to the new methodologies. While old dogs certainly can learn new tricks, unfortunately many old dogs don't want to, preferring to stay with old tricks even when the applause dies. Moreover, the elaborate rationales that they can give you for the superiority of their old ways can be amazing indeed.

These are all reasons for the paradox mentioned above. Certainly, any competent IS professional bringing health informatics today to a relatively uncomputerized hospital certainly would not start with obsolete software or hardware technologies and then scramble to catch up.

Accentuating this technical competency issue is the failure of many institutions to establish long-term or strategic IS policies. Rather, they vacillate over periods of time depending typically upon the personalities of the players involved. As an example, any institution needs to establish where it wants—and needs—to be on the technical innovation curve shown in Figure 1.1. Being at the far right, the leading edge of the leading edge, is a daring position, to say the least. In the informatics profession, this is often known as the "bleeding edge." The costs and the risks are extremely high, but so are the rewards in terms of system capabilities. This strategy can also appeal to the techies for its résumé value and its ego value at technical conventions. Few institutions can justify this pioneering approach, given the perils that befall most pioneers.

As one moves leftward, e.g., to the trailing edge of the leading edge, the risks and costs fall a bit as do the capability potentials. Most institutions, of course, fall into the broad middle range of balancing the variables involved. Normally, the left end of the curve is also a dangerous place to be. While risks and costs are low, so are

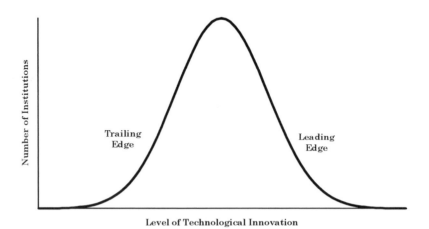

Figure 1.1. Schematic frequency distribution of the degree of aggressiveness in introducing technology into organizations.

the capabilities, with all the danger that brings to the overall institutional performance. As an example, many governmental agencies in the United States traditionally fell well to the left on this curve. The situation improved only after a number of changes were made such as in purchasing policies and practices.

When an organization fails to establish and follow a viable long-run technology strategy, the risk of implementation failures is raised significantly. The demands for staff competency are erratic, and the motivation of the technical work force typically varies widely as people are given challenges significantly above or below their competencies.

A final competency aspect is the technical competency of vendors and consultants. The further we press the competencies of our own staff, the more we must rely upon vendors and consultants. The IS area is notorious for having vendors that "blow in your ear and promise you anything!" The term *vaporware* was coined to describe the overwhelming number of grossly exaggerated promises made to prospective customers. Similarly, vendor employees often do not have the level of technical competence needed to supply the level of support promised during the sales process. The competency issue should not be as difficult to deal with in working with consultants if solid "hiring " practices are actually used, e.g., extensive reference checking. The challenge again arises when an extensive technology jump is involved, and we know so little about the area that we are unable to do much besides check references.

There is no question that technical competency will always be an issue in any highly technical, rapidly changing area. On the other hand, it is equally important to realize that technical competence is a necessary but not sufficient condition for implementation success.

Project Management Shortcomings

People who are highly trained technically—regardless of the technical area—are typically not renowned for the level of their management skills. Certainly, there are exceptions; however, the very attributes that make a person a good technician may well not be the attributes necessary for a good manager. Over the years, countless IS departments have developed the unfortunate reputation that every project takes twice as long, costs twice as much, and delivers half of what was promised.

We are using the term *project management* to refer to the internal management of the informatics project. All projects are defined in terms of three variables:

- ♦ *Scope*—the detailed specification of that to be accomplished as the project outcome.
- ♦ *Time*—the specific commitment to a date by which the scope will be completed.
- ♦ *Budget*—the budgeted resources of all types necessary to accomplish the scope by the specified date.

Managing significant health informatics projects is a challenging task. Typically, there are many uncertainties involved that make it difficult to accurately plan and estimate resources. There are many tools available to assist in project management such as work breakdown structures, linear responsibility charts, critical path methods (CPM), program review and evaluation techniques (PERT), etc. More important, in recent years it has become much easier to use these tools through inexpensive user-friendly micro-based computer software. One of the key benefits of this software is the ability to easily update the project plan, thereby maintaining a *dynamic* planning process throughout the project. In this era, it is inexcusable to attempt to manage a significant health informatics project without using advanced project management tools and software. Still, we see it frequently happening.

Organizational Shortcomings

As the quantity of biomedical knowledge has increased exponentially in recent years, informatics professionals have developed technical tools and strategies to cope with the vast volume and flow of information. These technical tools and strategies are constantly becoming more sophisticated, affecting more and more aspects of the biomedical organizations in which the strategies are implemented. These changes, often rapid, typically cause significant organizational stress.

Unfortunately, these organizational impacts are often not well understood by health informatics professionals. The impacts and the managerial strategies for dealing with them are typically not as easily defined and measured as their more technical counterparts.

It has become obvious in recent years that successfully introducing major new systems into complex organizations requires an effective blend of good technical and good organizational skills. The technically best system may be woefully inadequate if its implementation is resisted by people who have low psychological ownership in that system. On the other hand, people with high ownership can make a technically mediocre system function fairly well.

The Requirements for Systems Success

There are many ways to view systems depending upon the particular aspect being examined. In terms of the *components* of a health informatics system, we think of it as having three general components as shown in Figure 1.2.

Traditionally, the focus has been first on hardware, then on software, and finally on the "peopleware." Factors such as high out-of-pocket costs, high visibility, etc., have reinforced this hierarchy. The effect of this approach has been—and continues to be—that the *tools are stressed more than the product.* The typical result is systems that attempt to focus on and optimize processes rather than outcomes. For example, look at the traditional departmental title, "Data Processing." Unfortunately, changing the name of the department to "Information Systems" does not necessarily change the mind-set any more than changing the name of a traditional personnel department to "Human Relations" necessarily does.

To create quality systems, we need to look at three sets of skills shown in Figure 1.3—all of which are essential to a successful systems implementation. Where Figure 1.2 looked at the *components* of the system, Figure 1.3 looks at the *skills* involved in creating that system and its components.

Key System Components

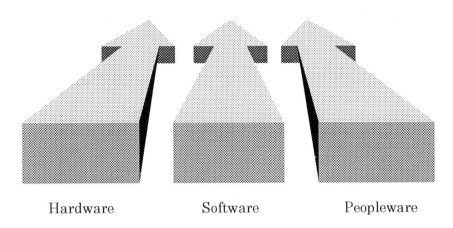

Hardware   Software   Peopleware

Figure 1.2. The key components of a successful health informatics implementation.

Making Systems Work

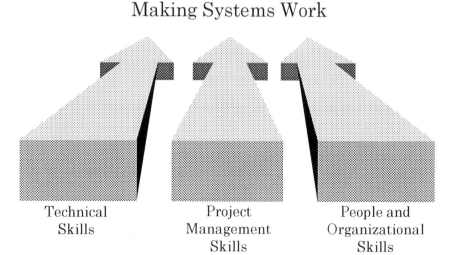

Technical	Project	People and
Skills	Management	Organizational
	Skills	Skills

Figure 1.3. The key skills necessary to create a successful health informatics implementation.

Technical skills include a broad range of skills, such as computer, telecommunications, medical, etc. This is the body of detailed technical knowledge, experience, and abilities—regardless of area—necessary to create a successful system. What are the structural requirements for a valid relational database? What are the necessary data elements for a patient record? Both of these questions arise in building a patient record database; however, the areas of technical expertise underlying the answers are very different.

Project management skills include the knowledge, techniques, and skills necessary for the successful internal management of significant information systems projects. Under this umbrella fall the traditional management functions such as planning, directing, controlling, motivating, and staffing. A good project manager must typically possess a blend of technical experience and managerial knowledge. From the technical side comes the ability to make accurate resource estimates, assign staff wisely, assist in problem solving, etc. From the managerial side comes the ability to do good planning, use project management models, motivate staff effectively, etc.

People and organizational skills include the wide range of skills necessary to effectively interface with all of the information system stakeholders outside the project team. A significant health informatics project typically has impacts on a wide range of people such as physicians, nurses, other members of the health care team, support staff, administrators, patients, vendors, etc. To ensure success, those spearheading the project must have a good level of skills at both the people or individual level and at the organizational or group level. A health informatics implementation can only be as successful as its ability to meet the often conflicting needs of these various stakeholders. It is through these people and organizational skills that the implementers determine these needs, build support for their work, and negotiate solutions to problems and conflicts.

The health informatics community has been slow to recognize the importance of these people and organizational skills. However, as implementation experiences have accumulated, more voices have been raised questioning the traditional technically dominated approach. For example, as Duke University worked its way through the Integrated Academic Information Management Systems (IAIMS) process, the leaders "learned that policy formulation and the ongoing planning aspects of the IAIMS model were more important then the technical aspects. Institutions will change, and an IAIMS must be dynamic enough to adapt."[3]

Why Haven't People and Organizational Issues Received Their Due?

Even when a sound approach to organizational issues contributes to good implementation results, the reaction often is, "Must have had great technical people on that project." Another common comment is that all that organizational stuff is "just common sense." When this type of comment comes from the techies—whether information systems or medical—part of it can probably be attributed to the common ego defense of discounting those attributes that we lack. However, there are a number of identifiable reasons why many tend to discount the areas of people and organizational skills.

Visibility

Hardware has a definite physical substance to it, even if we are only looking at pictures in a catalog. Even software can be physically represented by pictures of reports or computer screens. Organizational issues do not have this same physical visibility, especially in advance of true crises such as half the work force going on strike. We usually do not have a vivid organizational image equivalent to the Luddites destroying the hated factory machinery.

Measurability

Along with visibility, hardware and software also have a far higher degree of measurability, at least on certain dimensions. The hardware literature virtually buries us in numeric specifications while the software literature lists countless specific features. The costs (out-of-pocket only, of course) are also supposedly very specific. Again, those virtually invisible organizational issues are difficult to measure to any similar degree of firmness. We may know that the impact was significant, but there is no analogy to megabytes or milliseconds.

Predictability

The specifics of organizational issues are typically quite difficult to predict because they vary based upon the complex reactions of individuals and groups. While these reactions may be fairly predictable to the experienced professional, the predictability appears weak compared with the more visible and measurable hardware and software areas. A large part of this seemingly higher predictability may be illusory. Still, management is often far more comfortable allocating resources to areas with *seemingly* firmer data. At the same time, management may even be receiving glib predictions from the techies, "The users will love it!"

Accountability

Handling organizational issues or problems would seem to fall within the normal responsibilities of the managers of the various areas. The manager is supposed to be the "expert" in handling people. In reality, managers at the operating levels have often achieved their positions primarily through technical achievement and expertise and may be completely inept at managing major organizational change. Still, they may resist admitting their weaknesses or allowing outside experts to trod on their turf. On the other hand, these managers might welcome help but be afraid to ask and admit weakness. Senior management may see no problems ahead—the difficulty of prediction—or they may sincerely believe, "That's what we pay our managers for!"

Respectability

To people with technical and scientific backgrounds, the area of organizational issues is a fuzzy one filled with people with "soft-science" backgrounds. Even worse, many of these organizational experts have degrees called "interdisciplinary," which is a foreign concept to those who have risen through *traditional* academic channels. When some of the processes of organizational development and change management are described to these technical and scientific people, they often respond, "But that's just common sense," despite the fact that they don't exercise much of that so-called common sense in their organizations. At the extreme, the processes and techniques are deprecated as "touchy-feely" time wasters.

Timeliness

Conducting organizational processes such as extensive planning at the beginning of an information systems project is often regarded as delaying the "real work." In seminars, we jokingly refer to planning as an "un-American activity." Americans want to *do*! Nothing is happening until we are moving dirt! We are not making progress until we are writing code! In fact, this characteristic seems to apply to technical people in almost all the western cultures. To many techies, organizational processes seem to move at glacial speed with endless meetings and discussions about irrelevant topics such as *feelings*! This time factor alone accounts for significant resistance to more use of sound organizational processes.

Traditional Approach

What has been the traditional approach to organizational and people issues? First, when these issues have been considered at all, the focus has usually been limited to the hands-on users even though there may be many more stakeholders in the total information system. Second, the concern for these users often arises late in the project when someone says, "Oh yes, the users . . ." The concerns and needs of these users have often been a last-minute thought. Many technical decisions affecting the users often have already been made with little or no user input. Unfortunately, making meaningful changes in the system at this point is often prohibitively expensive.

The most common approach has been to focus on training as the answer to the end users' needs. There is no question that training is and will continue to be essential for the introduction of health informatics systems. Unfortunately, huge amounts of money have been wasted on inappropriate or low-quality training. Some of the typical shortcomings are:

- The recognition of the training need comes late in the process. The training is regarded as a low-status activity and is handed off to those low on the pecking order.
- The training design is often amateurish with the content not relevant to the users' real needs.
- Supervisors and managers are often not included in the training, leading to misunderstandings about the new system's quality and capabilities—or lack thereof.
- The training is often not professionally done, resulting in boring, ineffective training sessions.
- The amount of training—especially when physicians are involved—is often quite inadequate for true understanding of the new system.
- The training is often given too early, so that the learning is lost by the time that implementation actually occurs, or too late, so that untrained people have to struggle with the system.

System documentation and other ongoing user support aids have suffered from similar problems. Traditionally, documentation has also been an "afterthought" activity held in low esteem by the developers of the system. The preparation of documentation and other support tools has often been done at the end of a project while the technical people are eager to start on—or have already started—another technical project they find more professionally rewarding. Only in recent years has document preparation started to achieve a professional status of its own with a resulting significant increase in quality.

The Focus of This Book

As outlined earlier, a successful health informatics implementation requires sound skills in three areas: technical skills, project management skills, and organizational and people skills. Although all three are certainly critical, this book focuses on the area of organizational and people skills. This includes the practical implementation strategies necessary to make the system an operational success. However, health informatics implementations have a Heisenberg-type effect of their own. Once the new information system is implemented, the organization itself is changed. Therefore, a second aspect of this book is the recognition of those organizational changes and the adoption of strategies that will be effective in managing the altered organization.

Conclusion

Many health informatics implementations are less than completely successful. In some cases, the systems have not been outright failures but have failed to meet the user expectations. Based upon our studies, we know that these failures can be attributed to a combination of technical shortcomings, project management shortcomings, and organizational shortcomings. All of these shortcomings lead to stress and change-resistive behaviors. The next chapter presents some of the organizational change issues that the leaders of a health information system implementation must address.

Questions

1. How would you "cost out" an information system if you were to include many of the less tangible factors such as the people and organizational issues?
2. What is your opinion as to why information system failures happen?
3. What factors do you think a given institution should consider in positioning itself on the technological innovation curve shown in Figure 1.1?
4. Why do you think the people and organizational issues of health information systems have not received more attention in the past?

References

1.   Williams, LS. Microchips versus stethoscopes: Calgary hospital MDs face off over controversial computer system. *Can Med Assoc J* 1992;10:1534–1547.
2.   Dean, M. News: London perspective: Unhealthy computer systems. *Lancet* 1993;341:1269–1270.

3.   Stead, WW, Bird, WP, Califf, RM, et al. The IAIMS at Duke University Medical Center: Transition from model testing to implementation. *MD Computing* 1993;10:225–230.

2
Stress and Change Management in Implementing Health Informatics

This book is intended as a useful guide for managers of all types in the health care arena who face the challenge of introducing *significant informatics changes* into their organizations. It is impossible to introduce such a system into an organization without the people in that organization feeling the impact of change. The word *information* itself implies change since data become information only after the data are processed, i.e., altered, in ways that make the data useful for decision making. Inevitably, those enhanced decision making capabilities are going to affect the organization. People in the organization will often perceive effects such as:

- the pressure to develop new skills,
- the danger of looking stupid or incompetent in these new skill areas,
- loss of professional status,
- the pressure of higher performance expectations,
- the pressure of higher accountability through better measurements, and
- the danger of losing one's job to increasing automation.

Given these sorts of perceptions—real or imagined—it is under-standable that people may react quite adversely to the new system. If we are going to achieve successful implementations, we must have a solid understanding of change and change management processes.

The Relationship of Stress and Change

In the 1949 film of Graham Greene's novel *The Third Man*, Orson Welles as Harry Lime spoke the following words (which he had also written for the script): "In Italy for thirty years under the Borgias they had warfare, terror, murder, bloodshed—they produced Michelangelo, Leonardo da Vinci, and the Renaissance. In

Switzerland they had brotherly love, five hundred years of democracy and peace, and what did they produce? The cuckoo clock." Perhaps Welles was being a bit hard on the Swiss, but his point is clear: significant progress tends to require significant stimuli.

In that perfect world that none of us will ever see, all of our organizations—headed by dedicated, brilliant, and progressive leaders—would constantly strive for excellence independent of any external pressures. In the real world, the impact of inertia is huge. If not pressured, both organizations and individuals will tend to continue doing what they currently do—or very near derivatives of what they do. The phrase *comfort zone* is often used to describe this phenomenon.

To paraphrase the great stress expert, Dr. Hans Selye, we can view the absence of stress as death! At reasonable levels, stress is a potentially positive force for progress, an energizer for change. How well an individual or an organization handles a given stressor is often based upon the talent, experience, and self-esteem that are brought to the situation. Figure 2.1 shows the classical relationship between stress and productivity. Over a wide range, increasing levels of stress lead to higher productivity. However, a point is reached at which productivity begins to fall, often referred to as the point at which stress becomes distress. These first declines in productivity are often the result of errors of omission and/or commission.

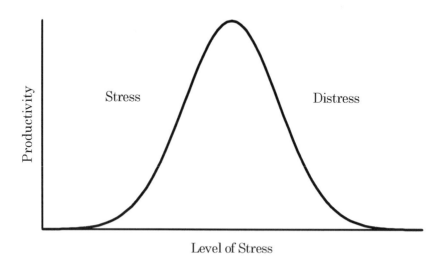

Figure 2.1. The relationship of levels of stress to levels to productivity.

There are three major strategies to follow when facing stress:

- avoid the stress,
- seek the stress, or
- manage the stress.

Avoiding stress is a sheeplike strategy that is usually suicidal over time in a dynamic environment. Constant avoidance of stressors normally leads to the birth and growth of even larger stressors—the old "molehills into mountains" effect. On the other hand, people who constantly seek stress have a death wish. Therefore, intelligent change managers are those who *manage* stress well in their approach to the change management process.

Stages in System Improvement

Figure 2.2 shows the stages of a typical health informatics implementation process. The stages are as follows:

- *Discontent*—the growing awareness that the existing system or method is unsatisfactory in meeting current or projected needs. This awareness may vary widely among the various organizational subgroups involved.
- *Conceptualization*—the analysis of the needs, analysis of the conflicting forces involved, and the broad design of the new system.
- *Planning*—the preparation of the implementation plan including detailed system specifications, timing, and resources.
- *Development*—the actual creation of the new operational system. This would typically be the longest of the stages in the creation of the new system.
- *Testing*—the testing and debugging of the system, typically a difficult balance between testing effectiveness and intrusiveness on ongoing operations.
- *Cutover*—the moment of truth when the system is put into operational use. In some cases, this may be a staged process, e.g., ward by ward. In other cases, circumstances may force an all-at-once or "suicide mission"-type conversion.

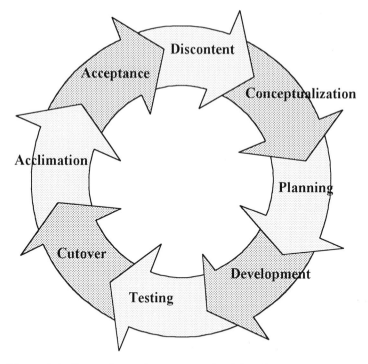

Figure 2.2. Stages in implementing a health informatics system.

- *Acclimation*—the period immediately after cutover in which the users receive their first live—as opposed to training—exposure to the new system. At the same time, the new information system receives its first exposure to the virtually infinite range of unpredicted demands, exceptions, etc.
- *Acceptance*—the period in which the system becomes and remains the new "way we have always done things around here." There are typically ongoing minor modifications or updates to the system during this acceptance period, which may well last for years for a quality system.
- *Discontent*—As the environmental forces change in various ways, the system starts to display inadequacies that start the process over again.

Notice that the process is depicted as a circle to convey its continuous nature. Discontent with the status quo is both the beginning of a cycle and its ultimate outcome. This discontent may reflect either external or internal pressures, i.e., stresses for change. Once begun, the change process itself becomes a potential source of stress to the organization with the highest stress typically occurring when the cutover is made to the new system. However, depending upon the initial "mental health" of the organization and the skill with which the change process is managed, the stress levels can be high or low at almost any stage.

Levels and Types of Change

What is a major change? A minor one? The magnitude of a change or a stressor—like beauty—is in the eye of the beholder. The proposed change that virtually terrorizes one person may be a welcome alleviation of boredom to the person in the next cubicle. Also, the types and magnitudes of reaction are often difficult for an "outsider" to predict. When working with change and change management, it often helps to have some ways of classifying the types and sizes of change.

A Model to Describe Levels of Change

Watzlawick et al.[1] have identified two levels of change:

- *First-order change* is a variation in the way processes and procedures have been done within a given system, leaving the system itself relatively unchanged. Some examples are creating new reports, creating new ways to collect the same data, refining existing processes and procedures, etc.
- *Second-order change* occurs when the system itself is changed. This type of change usually occurs as the result of a strategic change or a major crisis such as a threat against system survival. Second-order change involves a redefinition or reconceptualization of the business of the organization and the way it is to be conducted. In the medical area, changing from a full paper medical record to a full electronic medical record would represent a second-order change, just as automated teller machines redefined the way that many banking functions are conducted worldwide.

These two orders of change represent extremes. First order involves doing better what we now do, while second order radically changes the core ways we conduct business or even the basic business itself. There is a middle level that seems to be missing from these two extremes. Golembiewski et al.[2] added another level of change. They defined *middle-order change* as lying somewhere between the extremes of first and second order change. Middle-order change "represents a compromise; the magnitude of change is greater than first order change, yet it neither affects the critical success factors nor is strategic in nature."2 An example of a middle-order change might be the introduction of an electronic mail system into an organization. There is an organization-wide impact, but there is no reconceptualization of the basic business. E-mail is more of a tool for operational and communications efficiency.

Just as the levels of change are graduated, the resulting resistance to these changes is typically graduated also. Table 2.1 describes the first-order change situation. Both the levels of change and the levels of resistance are mild. Many of the resistance examples could be described as grumbling as opposed to any real

First-Order Change	Typical Resistance Examples
Modest effect on the total organizations processes	"Whose idea was this? Nobody asked me."
Modest impact on people—could help their efficiency	"I have my own way, and I like it fine, thank you!"
Improves on "the way we do things"	"This is too complicated."
Driving force is higher efficiency	"I don't like the computer looking over my shoulder."
	"This is more work! I want more money."
	"Why didn't they give us some decent training on this?"
	"If this is so great, why aren't the managers using it?"
	"You can't teach old dogs new tricks!"
	"The people who developed this should have to sit here and use it all day."

Table 2.1. First-order change characteristics and typical resistance examples.

resistance. Some of the common resistors in the first-order change level vary with personality type.

Some personality types will welcome changes that they perceive will make their jobs easier while other personality types use their day-to-day work rituals to build their comfort zones. In the late 1960s, one unit in a medical center started to code all of their continuing medical education courses with ICD 9 codes. Even though these codes were never used and took a great deal of time to complete, the organization did not want to change the process as time passed because "we have always done it this way." The old process lasted through two directors. When a new director went to change the process, there was definite resistance to this change.

Middle-Order Change	Typical Resistance Examples
Driving forces are both effectiveness and efficiency Medium to high impact on those performing the changed processes Major changes in processes, but the basic nature of the business not changed Some jobs may be eliminated	All of those shown under *First-Order Change* plus: "Work isn't fun anymore. I just hope I can hold out until I can retire." "Shows what loyalty counts for around here. Fourteen years and I'm out the door." "I'm not going to stick my neck out and get it chopped off." "What happens to the patients if this system quits on us?" "I didn't go to nursing school to be a data entry clerk for doctors." "I'm going to put my resume out on the market and see what happens." "This isn't how MDs should be spending their time." "We'll see what the union has to say about this!" "I've got plenty of sick leave, and I'm going to use it."

Table 2.2. Middle-order change characteristics and typical resistance examples.

Table 2.2 depicts the middle-order change situation in which both the degree and impacts of the change have increased as well as the intensity of the resistance. At this level of change, we start to see the possibility of much more aggressive resistance, including the possibility of collusive actions. The "No OSCAR" buttons described in Chapter 1 would be an example of this collusive type of action.

Table 2.3 illustrates second-order change, the most serious type. Here many of the resistance factors show employee despair and bitterness. For all but the most confident employees, their basic security needs are seriously threatened, which accounts for the depth of the resistance.

The five most important words to an individual involved in any change process are, "How will this affect me?" This is true regardless of the level or degree of change or the person's organizational position. The most traumatic changes are obviously in the second-order change category, but one person might perceive changes in the first or middle order as more traumatic than another person might perceive a second-order change. One of the challenges for the change manager is successfully managing these perceptions. How the change manager implements the process of change can have a decided effect on the resistance factors.

Second-Order Change	Typical Resistance Examples
Major effect on the organization's processes, which often are completely changed	All of those shown under *First-Order Change* and *Middle-Order Change* plus:
Typically a high impact on people and how they spend their time	"They say I'm safe, but I'm getting out the first chance I get."
Changes the basic business	"They can't make us do this!"
Whole areas of the business are sold, merged, or abandoned	"I just can't take any more of this kind of stress."
Driving force is a strategic decision, perhaps in response to major crises or basic survival threats	"I'm too old to start all over!"

Table 2.3. Second-order change characteristics and typical resistance examples.

Microchanges and Megachanges

At the more casual level, a classification scheme that we have found useful is that of microchanges and megachanges, with no great attempt at elaborate definitions. As a first approximation, the following scheme can be used to differentiate between the two:

- *microchanges*—differences in degree
- *megachanges*—differences in kind.

Using an information system as an example, modifications, enhancements, improvements, and upgrades would typically be microchanges while a new system or a very major revision of an existing one would be a megachange. This scheme works surprisingly well in communicating within organizations as long as we remember that one person's microchange is another person's megachange.

Types of Change

Changes within an organization can often be identified as one of four types with the definite possibility of overlap between two or more:

- *operational*—changes in the way that the ongoing operations of the business are conducted such as the automation of a particular area,
- *strategic*—changes in the strategic business direction, e.g., moving from an inpatient to an outpatient focus,
- *cultural*—changes in the basic organizational philosophies by which the business is conducted, e.g., implementing a Continuous Quality Improvement (CQI) system,
- *political*—changes in staffing occurring primarily for political reasons of various types such as occur at top patronage job levels in government agencies.

These four different types of change typically have their greatest impacts at different levels of the organization. The following four figures illustrate this point.

Figure 2.3 shows that operational changes tend to have their greatest impacts at the lower levels of the organization, right on the firing line. Those at the upper levels may never notice changes that cause significant stress and turmoil to those attempting to implement the changes.

Figure 2.4 shows that changes in the organization's strategic direction have potentially significant impacts at all levels of the organization. Some similar activities will continue despite the changes; the accountants will still be doing financial reports, for example. Still, the nature and type of virtually everyone's work will be noticeably affected.

Figure 2.5 shows that cultural changes typically affect all levels but have their strongest impact on the middle levels. This phenomenon has occurred countless times in recent years as organizations have introduced cultural changes stressing values such as employee empowerment, open communications, etc. The traditional roles of those in the middle have been changed completely, calling for new skills, attitudes, and behaviors. This explains why resistance to cultural change has often been higher in the middle than at lower levels as many would expect if they have not been through such a change process.

Figure 2.6 shows that the impact of political changes is typically felt most at the higher organizational levels. As the name implies, these changes are typically not made for results-oriented reasons but for reasons such as partisan politics or internal power struggles. When these changes occur in a relatively bureaucratic organization —as they often do—the bottom often hardly notices the changes at the top. Patients are seen and the floors are cleaned exactly the same as before. The key point is that performance was not the basis of the change; therefore, the performers are not affected that much.

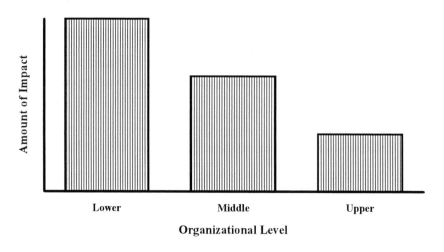

Figure 2.3. Impacts of operational changes by organizational level.

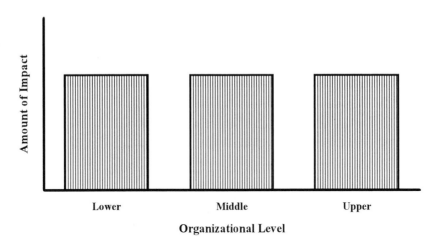

Figure 2.4. Impacts of strategic changes by organizational level.

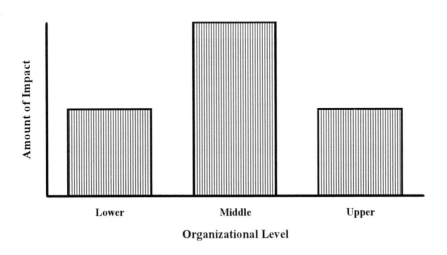

Figure 2.5. Impacts of cultural changes by organizational level.

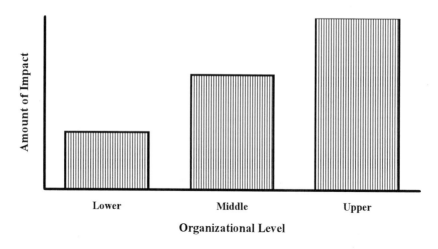

Figure 2.6. Impacts of political changes by organizational level.

Resistance to Change

It has been said that the only person who welcomes change is a wet baby! It seems to be part of the human makeup to be most comfortable with the status quo unless it is inflicting discomfort. Even then, people will often resist a *specific* change. This is probably the "devil you know is better than the devil you don't know" phenomenon. It is a shock for inexperienced managers the first time they see subordinates resist even a change that they requested.

Resistance Against What?

There can be countless reasons for resistance to change in a given situation, and the term *resistance to change* is often used very broadly. One of the first aspects that must be analyzed in a given situation is the difference between

- resistance to a particular *change* and
- resistance to the perceived *changer(s)*.

In the first case, the resistance is actually directed against the changes in the system. In the second case, the resistance occurs because of negative feelings toward the organization in general, specific units, or specific managers. In this second case, virtually any change would be resisted just because of who is perceived in favor of it. Both have to be dealt with, but it is critical that we identify the primary one we are facing.

When a new health informatics system is introduced, three factors are very important:

- ◆ What is the general organizational climate—positive or negative, cooperative or adversarial, etc.?
- ◆ What has been the quality of the *process* used to implement previous informatics systems?
- ◆ What has been the technical quality of the informatics systems previously implemented?

Even if we may be new to an organization, we inevitably inherit to some degree the organizational climate and history. Negative "baggage" of this type can be a frustrating burden that adds significantly to the challenge of successfully implementing a new system. On the other hand, the ability to meet this type of challenge is a differentiating factor for truly skilled implementers.

Intensity of Resistance

Resistance can vary from the trivial to the ferocious. Also, the very perception of resistance can vary widely from one observer to another. One might perceive an end user who asks many questions as being very interested and aggressively seeking knowledge. Another might see the same person as a troublemaker who should just "shut up and listen!"

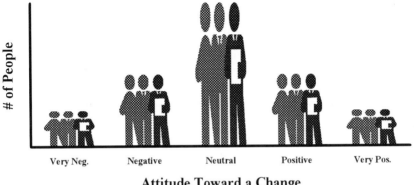

Attitude Toward a Change

Figure 2.7. An organization with a basically neutral attitude toward change.

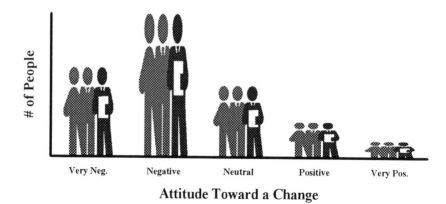

Attitude Toward a Change

Figure 2.8. An organization with a basically negative attitude toward change.

We can safely assume that every significant health informatics implementation is going to encounter some resistance; however, the intensity can vary widely. Figure 2.7 depicts a situation in which significant numbers of the people are initially neutral toward a particular proposed systems change. Overall, a definite majority of the people are neutral to positive about the change. At the same time, there is a definite negative component to be managed. This is not an atypical situation in an organization with decent morale and a history of managing changes reasonably well. The challenge here is to use sound organizational processes of the sort presented later in the book to overcome the negative factors. At the very least, this negative portion must be prevented from growing.

Figure 2.8 depicts a very different situation. Here, the proposed change faces a strong negative bias that could arise from various sources as discussed above. This is the high-challenge situation for systems implementers and it is unfortunately common.

If Figure 2.8 describes an implementer's hell, Figure 2.9 depicts sheer heaven. There is a high positive attitude toward the change with only a low portion having feelings of resistance. If Figure 2.9 represents an *initial attitude* toward the proposed change, a lot of things have been done right in the past in this organization. The general morale must be good and the aftertaste left by past systems implementations must be quite positive. We can think of Figure 2.9—or an even more positive distribution—as our goal as we progress in our current implementation. If the initial attitude we face is something like Figure 2.8, our work is cut out for us.

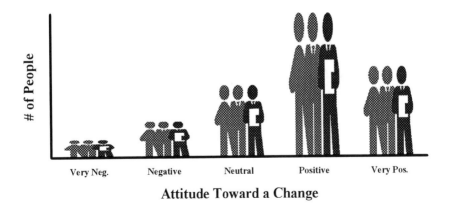

Figure 2.9. An organization with a basically positive attitude toward change.

Using These Models

Merely identifying the types and levels of change we face will not solve the change management challenges that we will encounter in implementing health informatics systems. However, it is a first step in organizing our thinking about these challenges. If we identify and define these change issues better, we will be able to use more effectively the change management strategies described later in this book. In the next chapter we will review some of the critical aspects affecting change management in today's health care environment. The remainder of the book will then present practical strategies and tactics for dealing with the issues raised in this chapter.

Conclusion

It is impossible to introduce a new technology-based system into an organization without the people in the organization feeling the impact of the change. The challenge to organizations is to acknowledge the stress that change will bring to both the people as individuals and the organization as a whole. In this chapter, we presented some of the issues of organizational change and resistance to change, which are common to virtually any organization. In the next chapter some of the unique issues encountered within the health care environment will be specifically addressed.

Questions

1. What are some typical signs of stress that an organization encounters when a major informatics system is implemented?
2. What are several first-order and second-order changes that you have personally experienced? Compare one of the first-order changes and one of the second-order changes in terms of the stress levels involved in each.
3. Of the four types of changes—operational, strategic, cultural, and political—which one is the most difficult to deal with and why? Least difficult and why?
4. What is the most dramatic example of resistance to change that you have ever encountered? Why was the change resisted so strongly? Looking back, what strategies might have been used to facilitate the change process?

References

1. Watzlawick, P, Weakland, JH, Fisch, R. *Change: Principles of Problem Formulation and Problem Resolution* New York:W.W. Norton, 1974.
2. Golembiewski, RT, Billingsley, K, Yeager, S. Measuring change and persistence in human affairs: Types of change generated by OD designs, *Journal of Applied Behavioral Science* 1976;12:133–157.

3
Today's Health Care Environment

Implementing major informatics systems in any organization—even in a so-called "computer" company—is a challenge. When we look at organizations with widely varying missions, there are still many common aspects. They are all staffed with people possessing the normal set of human frailties. There is often a basic set of administrative-type functions that have to be performed. At the same time, the specific missions of two seemingly similar health care organizations, e.g., two hospitals, might require significant differences in many of their information systems. The needs of a large urban trauma center might be quite different from those of a rural feeder hospital.

In this chapter we look first at some major changes in the general information environment and then specifically at the health care industry and some of its particular issues. Today, virtually all organizations are facing megachanges in their environments. In the past, the health care industry has been sheltered from many environmental forces, but this situation is rapidly ending. Those charged with implementing health informatics systems will be operating in a more and more dynamic environment over the coming decade.

Today's Changing Information Environment

From the time that our ancestors huddled in caves, every generation has probably complained about the massive changes it was facing. Whether the Dark Ages or the Industrial Revolution, the "present" seemed to be a time of high change for those living it. However, we strongly feel that history will show that we are living in one of those "revolutionary" eras rather than one of the more stagnant ones.

In 1964, Bob Dylan's song, "The Times They are A-Changing," emphasized the massive social changes occurring in the United States during that era. Yet for many organizations in the industrialized world, the truly massive changes did not start to occur for approximately another twenty years. Over the past decade, many organizations have felt the pressures for megachange, and our health care systems are now being drawn into this high-stress arena. Many European health care systems—facing figurative, if not literal bankruptcy—are looking at ways to slash costs. The United States health care system is facing huge unknown changes. Hospitals in the United States are already merging at near frantic rates. Some of these pressures are linked to larger structural forces acting on today's industrial nations, and those of us concerned about managing change in health care settings are heavily affected by these larger issues.

Unfortunately, when we feel we are trapped on the back of a tiger, we tend to do a lot of very short-run thinking! The stresses of the moment seem to demand our full attention. However, there are people studying the bigger picture who have some interesting insights to share—insights that may explain some of the more frightening aspects of today's megachanges. Paul A. David, a Stanford economic historian, has studied a paradox that has troubled many of us who have been involved with information systems for years: Where are the productivity gains from the billions of dollars we have poured into information technology over the past forty years? Further, is the computer revolution going to create a small, extremely well-paid elite, with the rest of us condemned to flipping hamburgers or cleaning each other's bathrooms?

David examines in economic detail the years from 1880 to 1920, a forty-year period over which the electrification of the industrialized world took place.[1] Despite the glowing promises of electrification, productivity increases during this period were minimal. (Does this sound familiar, computer users?) Why did this happen? The new technology was merely being applied to existing paradigms—organizational structures, market structures, legal frameworks, work force skills, etc. Further, the economic measures of productivity were unable to adequately measure product enhancements or improvements in quality—a problem that plagues us yet today. We still don't know how to measure the productivity gain of a *faster* trip on an electric train or of a treatment that is *less painful* to the patient. Put another way, the full benefits of a new technology are realized only as the total framework or paradigm slowly shifts to allow those full benefits to take effect. At the same time, the paradigm shifts might well not be possible without that new technology.

What does this mean for us in an organizational sense? The full benefits of information systems in our health care systems will accrue *only* after our health care systems have undergone massive transformations, which in turn could not have happened without these new information technologies. In health care, we are much closer to the beginning of these massive transformations than to the end!

Perhaps more important, what are the implications for more personal or human issues such as employment and real wages? In the industrial countries, we are experiencing significant "downsizing," "rightsizing," "rationalization," etc. Real wages seem to be stagnant or even declining. Even supposed "knowledge workers" are losing jobs. All this is very similar to what happened in the past when new economic paradigms arose.

Figure 3.1 shows in a schematic sense what occurs during these paradigm shifts. The *Old* curve represents the employment levels generated at a point in time by the old paradigm, while the *New* curve represents the same for the new paradigm—in this case the reconstructed *true information economy*. Until some point in time, the old economy sheds workers faster than the new aspects of the economy create *similar quality jobs*. The sum of these two employment curves is shown in Figure 3.2 with the minimum point occurring at the same time as the intersection of the two curves in Figure 3.1.[2]

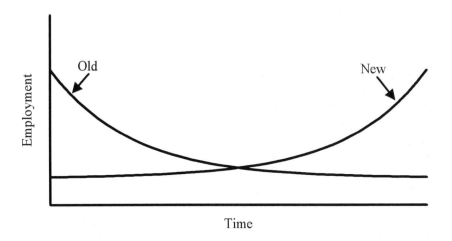

Figure 3.1. Employment levels provided by the old and new paradigms over time.

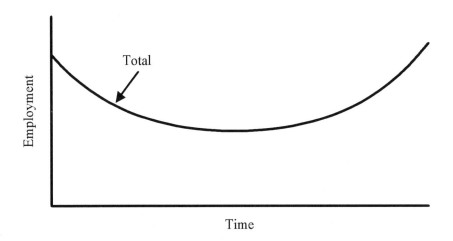

Figure 3.2. The total employment provided by both old and new paradigms over time.

When will this minimum point occur? Expert opinions vary; however, many believe that in the United States the bottom point on the Figure 3.2 curve will occur in the latter half of the 1990s, perhaps 1997 or 1998. In Europe, the situation is not so clear. European economies have traditionally focused more on job protection than on efficiency increases; therefore, the European economies have lagged in making some of their difficult downsizing decisions. Also, while private sector employment in the United States has increased by 50 percent since 1970, the net increase in Europe has been zero. All job growth—about 10 percent—has come in the public sector. In the meantime, until a resumption of job growth is perceived, many people will remain extremely nervous. We observed a recent merger of two hospitals; the overwhelming reaction of the two staffs was fear of job loss, even among physicians and nurses whose jobs were in little or no danger. The general feelings of uncertainty and insecurity about job loss are a definite factor that health care change managers will have to face more and more over the next decade.

When changes in information systems are part of other massive changes occurring within an organization, the potential for resistance is immense. The information system—being highly visible—may serve at times as a whipping boy for changes that are really organizational in nature. During the next decade, successfully overcoming resistance to change will be a key factor in achieving successful health informatics implementations.

How Health Care Organizations are Different

As stated earlier, health care organizations have a combination of attributes that makes them quite different from other types of organizations. While other organizations might possess a few of the differentiating attributes, most health care organizations possess a great majority of them. At the same time, health care organizations do share many characteristics with other organizations of similar size. We examine here some of both types of factors.

Different countries can have quite different health care structures. In the following discussion, we use the United States system as an example. Also, we use hospitals as our primary example of health care organizations because of the size and complexity of these organizations and their informatics systems.

Life-and-Death Issues

Hospitals deal continuously with life-and-death issues. Errors of either omission or commission can lead to serious harm to real people. Moreover, this harm is not in the abstract sense of someone a thousand miles away being killed by faulty product design or manufacture five years later. When a Chilean futures trader entered "sell" instead of "buy" into his computer terminal, it may have cost his organization over $30 million, but nobody died from it.[3] Hospital errors can mean first having to watch the tragedy, then having to console the survivors, and, perhaps most difficult, having to live with the feeling of responsibility or possibly even guilt. This life- and-death responsibility constantly affects health care processes and procedures, leading to significant differences from other organizations involved in less dramatic activities. At the same time, we must recognize that the banner of "patient care" has been waved countless times in hospital settings to justify needless expenditures or purchases that were actually desired for reasons of ego, status, convenience, etc. Still, when working with health care information systems, we have to be constantly aware of the risk management issue in terms of expending ample resources at all stages to ensure extremely high accuracy on issues involving patient health. We want all our systems to be accurate, but we can tolerate billing or payroll errors far easier than we can tolerate errors in clinical systems.

Complex Personnel Structure

Hospitals have a very complex personnel structure, using "personnel" here in a broad sense. Normally, an organization's staff is made up of employees, supplemented perhaps by so-called temps or people working on contract. Regardless of the type, the organization does have direct control over the behaviors of these employees or quasi-employees. In a simplistic sense, the organization ultimately could tell the people to "shape up or ship out" if they display too much resistance to the change. According to George Anders of the *Wall Street Journal*, "But unlike big corporations, where top management can issue orders to its employees, hospital executives must delicately sell these strategies to hundreds of largely independent doctors. The physicians have final authority in deciding how to treat a patient. And at many teaching hospitals, top doctors earn more and are far more renowned than even the institution's chief executive."[4]

The majority of the physicians, who are the dominant force in the health care delivery process, are typically not employees of the hospital. In fact, these physicians often provide to the hospital many of its patients—especially the acute-care ones. If the physicians have alternative hospitals they can recommend to their patients, the physicians are in a position of high power. Historically, many hospitals have aggressively wooed their local physicians in an attempt to generate additional business.

As more and more clinical informatics projects are implemented, the support—or at least acquiescence—of these physicians is critical. This in turn places high pressure on the informatics implementers to avoid harming the relationships between the physicians and the hospital. We should note, however, that even in cases in which the physicians are employees, the problem of the power of physicians and other health professionals can be significant. This type of problem can arise whenever employees have significantly higher allegiance to their professions than to their employer. Health care professionals certainly tend to have this type of strong feelings and are typically quick to rebel at anything that they perceive will harm either the quality of patient care or the status and discretionary powers of their profession.

Alternative Ownership Characteristics

Hospitals in the United States have a wide array of alternative ownership characteristics. Some hospitals are parts of extensive "chains" of one sort or another, while others are stand-alone units.

Some are for-profit with profit objectives similar to those of for-profit businesses, but the great majority are some form of not-for-profit organization. Within this broad not-for-profit category, some of the hospitals are owned and operated by various governmental entities, some by religious or fraternal based organizations, and some by not-for-profit corporations established solely for the purpose of creating a hospital.

The for-profit hospitals have typically been criticized—justly or unjustly—for doing only those things that contribute to their profits, i.e., "skimming" the market, leaving the unprofitable activities to be handled by the not-for-profit hospitals operating under more altruistic motives. The for-profits have responded that the not-for-profits have operated for years in grossly inefficient manners lacking any motivation to improve. This is not the arena to settle that debate; however, it can safely be said that any pursuit of excellence in the not-for-profits has typically had to come from within the hospitals themselves as their boards of directors normally contain little or no health care management expertise. Board members have often been selected either for their abilities to donate or raise funds or as representatives of major employers in the area. In the latter case, these representatives are typically executives in areas such as human resources, public relations, or community relations, not in operating areas. These boards do choose the senior hospital leadership; however, the boards then have little internal expertise with which to judge the performance of that leadership. The point here is that optimal leadership strategy is often a defensive rather than an offensive one. Avoiding risks and problems can tend to have a higher value than making incisive forward-looking decisions, especially ones that involve high profile risk.

Many and Varied Stakeholders

Just as hospitals are different in personnel and ownership characteristics, they are different in terms of their many and varied stakeholders. This difference also extends in general to the entire health care area. Among these many stakeholders, the needs, desires, attitudes, etc., can vary widely, presenting many potential conflict situations for health care leaders to resolve. The stakeholders for a typical hospital might include

- the owning entity or group,
- the general public,
- various levels of government,
- vendors,

+ the professional staff,
+ the other staff members,
+ physicians with admitting privileges,
+ patients,
+ families of patients,
+ third-party payers or payment administrators, and
+ area employers.

It is hard to conceive of a non–health care for-profit company having a set of stakeholders anywhere near this complicated.

Declining Public Image

In the "good old days," the entire health care profession enjoyed a rather exalted status. The kindly family doctor made house calls at all hours and sometimes received only a chicken or a baby pig in payment. Florence Nightingale roamed the halls with her lamp, alleviating suffering as she went. These professionals were regarded as wonderful humans doing the best they could. Patients understood that treatments involved risks, and that the professionals occasionally would make mistakes. While patients would not always do what the doctors said, their instructions were generally unquestioned. Hospitals were similarly regarded. Everyone complained about the food, but the general image was quite positive.

Things are different today for a variety of reasons too complex to analyze here. Perfect outcomes are demanded, regardless of the risks involved. It is an era of cynicism and malpractice suits. Anyone designing and implementing health informatics systems today has to realize these potential implications. The systems must not only perform well, they must have the *image* of performing well. Systems must not rely on human interventions to avoid treatment errors. Low consequence faults in a system can still be used by others to cast doubts on a system's quality. Errors in billing, for example, can be used to cast doubts about the quality of clinical systems. Further, systems must include extensive audit trails to ensure that it can be *proven* that appropriate actions were taken in given circumstances. In today's adversarial legal environment, health informatics systems must do their share in implementing a philosophy of protecting against after-the-fact criticisms.

Exploding Technologies

Since World War II, health care technology has exploded in terms of both knowledge and hardware. In a private conversation, an elderly world-famous physician recounted to us the frustrations of her early days in medicine. For many patient problems that are treated routinely today, the physician in those days could only serve as a hand holder, hoping to make the end easier for the patient and the family. Contrast this with the comments of C. K. Meador, a Vanderbilt University physician, who observes that well people are vanishing and predicts the extinction of the "species" will occur in late 1998. His point is that a public obsessed with complete and definitive "wellness"—combined with ever more powerful clinical diagnostic technologies—can find *something wrong with everyone.*[5] These technologies extend to the treatment side as well as the diagnostic side. Premature babies are saved at stages considered impossible ten years ago. Transplant operations of various types are routinely successful. Today's experimental procedures become tomorrow's routine.

Paralleling this explosion in clinical technology is the explosion in medical information in both print and electronic form. The challenge facing medical informatics is the effective integration and dissemination of all the clinical data with this medical information along with other informatics tools such as decision support systems. Further, all this must be done in a way that is flexible enough to accommodate unknown future developments in these exploding areas.

Rising Costs

The pressure of rising health care costs is being felt in all the industrialized countries today. These countries are typically spending somewhere *between 7 and 14 percent* of their gross domestic products on health care. This means that health care is both a massive cost to these countries and a significant part of their economies in terms of employment, construction, sales of equipment and supplies, etc. General Motors most significant vendor is not the steel industry, it is Blue Cross/Blue Shield.

Unless artificially restrained, health care costs tend to steadily rise, with the pressures for increase including

- the exploding technologies discussed above,
- aging populations,
- rising patient expectations,

- general inflationary pressures,
- legal liability issues, and
- the practice of "defensive medicine."

In the United States, hospital bills of $250,000 or more, while not common, are certainly not rare. While various strategies can be used to contain or even reduce these overall health care costs on a temporary basis, the only way to contain costs in the long run is by some form of either rationing or strong price controls, however they are implemented.

The challenge in implementing health informatics in increasingly cost conscious environments will be to include cost considerations in two ways:

1. designing and implementing systems in cost-effective ways and
2. designing systems that integrate financial and nonfinancial data in ways that support sound financial decision making by everyone in all areas at all levels.

Oligopolistic Economic Environment

In the health care arena, hospitals have traditionally practiced very little, if any, price competition. Hospitals have typically found themselves in near-monopolistic or oligopolistic market situations and have behaved accordingly. An oligopolistic market is one with a few large producers, each having a significant market share. Oligopolistic organizations typically avoid price competition if at all possible because the potential outcome is bitter price wars that turn out to be harmful to all. If possible, they engage in explicit or implicit price fixing and then "compete" vigorously in areas such as the advertising of "unique" features. A typical example would be aggressively advertising their maternity service as being the "best" in some noncontroversial way such as having beautiful new facilities or providing tender loving care. Advertising infant mortality rates would be taboo as it would invite aggressive reprisal.

An outcome of this limited type of competition is that most hospitals have sparse managerial financial data compared with many for-profit organizations. It is a rare hospital that can provide meaningful cost data that are useful in a managerial sense. In addition, many hospitals have traditionally engaged in so much cost shifting from one segment of their population to another for political reasons that they prefer that truly accurate information remains unknown.

As the health care systems in all countries come under increasing economic pressures, health informatics systems will have to provide better financial data in a managerial sense, integrating modern techniques such as activity-based costing into the managerial information systems.

Unique Payment Structure

One of the significant characteristics of the health care structure in the United States—at least historically—is the source of payments for medical care. In the typical economic transaction, the recipient of the goods or services pays for them after making a judgment that the value of what is to be received is greater than the value of what is to be given in exchange. The very nature of the health care model starts to distort this basic model for at least two reasons:

1. in many cases, the recipient of the services, i.e., the patient, has not anticipated needing the services and is not in a mental or physical condition to do comparison shopping, and
2. the patient may have limited input into the choice of a hospital either because of physician influence, emergency conditions, or limited options.

Further, hospitals typically provide only very limited information to incoming patients about costs, e.g., only room charges, leading to an uninformed economic choice.

All of the above implies that the patient would even care about the cost. Over the past fifty years, encouraged by the tax code, a system has evolved in the United States that has isolated the majority of patients from the payment process so effectively that many patients never even see the hospital bill. The payment of the bill by private insurers or employer funds has further distorted this economic transaction. Patients often have little or no incentive to care about—let alone to help control—the costs of their health care. Faced with exploding costs, third-party payers have tried various schemes over the past decade to instill in the patients a sense of the costs of their health care, and these schemes have met with varying success. When health care is provided by a governmental system, the same general problems apply. The decision processes that govern our normal economic lives simply do not apply in the health care area.

Strong Traditional Roles and Ethical Codes

The health care industry contains many professional groups such as physicians, nurses, pharmacists, etc., each of which has a traditional role in the system and a strong ethical code. For example, a common expression of the values that govern medical ethics is beneficence, nonmaleficence, autonomy, veracity, justice, and confidentiality. What do these mean in practice? How might they affect the design of a system, if at all? Any implementation of health informatics systems has to consider these issues.

What might seem to be an obviously desirable change for the sake of efficiency or simplicity might be organizationally disastrous. Moreover, when such changes are implemented by other parts of the organization, the informatics systems may unfortunately inherit the whipping boy role as the systems may be the most visible physical manifestations of the changes.

Complex Confidentiality Issues

Hospitals—and their information systems—have to deal with complex confidentiality issues. All organizations have to deal with confidentiality issues such as personnel records. Some have more complex issues such as trade secrets or government security requirements. However, hospitals face a difficult challenge in adequately protecting patient confidentiality while affording sufficient information access to ensure quality care. Further, errors in either direction can expose the hospital to significant legal liability. In research-oriented institutions, there is often an additional problem of providing adequate information access for research purposes while still protecting the confidentiality of patients.

Regulatory and Accreditation Requirements

Hospitals operate under a very complex set of regulatory and accreditation requirements that puts special demands upon the information systems for the maintenance of adequate records in appropriate form. Further, the systems must have the flexibility to accommodate new regulations or reporting requirements that can arise at any time.

How Health Care Organizations are Not Different

Hospitals are complex organizations made up of a wide variety of subsystems. Some of these subsystems are quite similar to those found in other organizations. For example, payroll systems with all their complexities are quite similar for virtually all organizations of similar sizes. Those systems more closely linked to administrative processes share commonalties with nonhospital systems. It is the systems linked closely to the clinical processes that are relatively unique. This point is important because quite sophisticated work has been done in some areas in nonhospital systems, e.g., personnel scheduling, inventory control, personnel systems, maintenance management, numerous accounting functions, etc. It is critical that hospital systems build upon this accumulated knowledge where appropriate rather than simply computerizing traditional hospital procedures and processes. Further, there is no assurance that some of the "integrated" hospital information systems make use of the more sophisticated approaches in some of their modules.

The application of general models to the hospital setting can at least make us examine our traditional assumptions on the best ways to run the system. For example, a hospital can be viewed as a job-shop type facility with the patients being the work-in-process inventory. (We wouldn't necessarily want to share this viewpoint with the patients!) Why do this? Many tools have been developed for optimizing job-shop operations through the identification of process bottlenecks.[6] Even if we decide not to adopt a particular strategy for some reason, e.g., employee morale, using such a model can often tell us what our decision is costing us.

As we design and refine our health informatics systems, it is critical that we capture the types of data that will enable us to utilize modern management tools that have often been developed in nonhospital areas. These data and analyses have the potential to show us far higher productivity gains than we will achieve by merely "tweaking" our current systems.

Some Current Environmental Forces

In addition to some of the pressures mentioned above such as cost containment or reduction, there are a variety of other forces and pressures at work on the health care area. As they affect various health care arenas and organizations, they will have an impact on the health informatics area.

Demands for Accountability and Outcomes Measurement

As resources become dearer, payers want assurance that their money is being spent on treatments that are both effective and efficient. Health care data traditionally have been activities oriented rather than outcomes oriented. Whole new ways of measuring, capturing, storing, and analyzing data are being aggressively developed.

Prevention Versus Treatment

As part of both the wellness and the cost reduction movements, there is an increasing emphasis on the prevention of medical problems rather than just the treatment. The cost/benefit ratio of this approach tends to make it a very intelligent approach. As an example, the tremendous increases in life expectancy that the world has experienced this century are far more attributable to public health achievements in the prevention of disease than to improved treatments of sick or injured patients.

Alternate Forms of Treatment

For various sociological reasons, there has been an increasing interest in alternative treatment forms, e.g., acupuncture, many of which were introduced from other cultures. In addition, the various holistic approaches fit with the emphasis on wellness mentioned above. As some of these approaches are integrated into the mainstream, health informatics will have to adapt to new information needs.

Shifting Management Paradigms

As the conventional paradigms for organizational interactions change in the general economy, health care institutions come under pressure to follow suit, regardless of their traditions. Godlike behavior by physicians or anyone else is tolerated less and less by today's work force. A few of the current trends are

- a desire for worker empowerment,
- a desire for higher job flexibility, and
- a demand for the recognition and respect of work force diversity.

Moreover, these trends show no signs of abating.

Implied Competitive Expectations

Although true competition among health care organizations is somewhat limited as discussed earlier, the general level of progress in an economy still has an impact on the expectations that people have for health care organizations. If one telephone call can correct my telephone bill, why do I have to call the doctor's office four times to get a billing error straightened out? Why can my dog's veterinarian look things up quickly on the computer while my doctor fumbles through a paper file? As people interact with various systems, they form a set of general expectations that they expect other systems to meet. This forms a definite challenge for health care institutions, which have traditionally put a significantly lower portion of revenues into the information systems area compared with businesses of comparable size.

As people see the philosophies and teachings of quality gurus such as Deming, Jurand, Crosby, Taguchi, and others put into effect in their own work places, they will increasingly expect the same levels of performance and quality from their health care providers.

Conclusion

This chapter has provided a quick overview of some of the peculiarities of the health care area. Ultimately, to gain the information and knowledge necessary for successful health informatics implementations, a person needs to

- ◆ spend time in the area,
- ◆ realize that health care organizations are not just like any other,
- ◆ be sensitive to the needs of both the organization and the people,
- ◆ ask questions and listen well, and
- ◆ follow the sound organizational and people practices laid out in the rest of this book.

The following two sections analyze the organizational and people issues the informatics implementer is going to encounter and provide some proven techniques for successful implementation.

Questions

1. What are your suggested strategies for individuals to prepare for competing in the true information economy?
2. What reasons do you see as to why hospitals are "different" types of organizations beside those listed in this chapter?
3. How would you rank hospitals, newspaper publishing companies, stock brokerage companies, and high-tech manufacturing companies with respect to being information- based organizations? Explain your rankings.
4. What are some other possible environmental forces that might affect various types of health care organizations?

References

1. David, PA. *Computer and Dynamo: The Modern Productivity Paradox in a Not-Too-Distant Mirror.* CEPR Pub. #172, Stanford Center for Economic Policy Research, 1989.
2. Riley, RT. Living through megachanges. *Organizational Issues in Medical Informatics* 1994;1(3):1–2.
3. Moffett, M. A typing brush-up might be in order for a "mad genius." *Wall Street Journal* March 16, 1994, A1–A14.
4. Anders, G. Require surgery: Health plans force even elite hospitals to cut costs sharply. *Wall Street Journal* March 8, 1994, A1–A8.
5. Meador, CK. The last well person. *New England Journal of Medicine* 1994;6:440–441.
6. Goldratt, EM, Cox, J. *The Goal: A Process of Ongoing Improvement,* revised edition. Croton-on-Hudson: North River Press, 1986.

Section II
Organizational Issues

Introduction

This section presents the organizational issues, strategies, and tools involved in implementing health informatics systems in today's health care environment.

Chapter 4 presents the role and implications of organizational culture, models of information politics, and organizational growth stages on the management of information technology resources.

Chapter 5 presents the key areas that must be considered in preparing the organization for the changes inherent in the systems implementation process.

Chapter 6 presents the development and refinement of an organization's strategic information technology plan. It includes guiding principles and a set of key questions that an organization must address as it creates its strategic direction.

Chapter 7 presents the key people and organizational issues in planning and managing a significant health informatics project. This includes the establishment of realistic performance expectations for both the implementation process and for system performance.

Chapter 8 presents the key elements essential to the management of those changes that are an inherent part of the implementation of significant health informatics systems.

Chapter 9 presents the organizational political issues and the strategies necessary to successfully negotiate the political minefields that surround the organization's information technology area.

4
Operating in Different Organizational Structures

Organizations are messy places! They are made up of people who bring widely varying personalities, values, and agendas into the organization. Many of us feel that truth, beauty, and justice should prevail, and then we find out that power prevails. All we should have to do is present our obviously brilliant idea or plan, and everyone should leap to their feet shouting their agreement, unless they are too awestruck by the brilliance, of course. In reality, we find that we have to constantly sell, negotiate, and compromise to get those ideas or plans approved.

To be successful, health informatics systems need to support—or at least not be in conflict with—the organizational structures of the organization in which the systems are implemented. Therefore, it is critical that the implementer analyzes and understands those structures. The plural is used because organizations and their subunits have multiple structures within structures. Organizations base their organizational operating structures on what they perceive will both meet their cultural and political needs and also be successful for them.

There are three basic types of health informatics organizational structures: centralized, decentralized, and matrix. The creation and maintenance of one of these structures is dependent on three supporting concepts, the organization's culture, the organization's political process, and the organization's stage of growth. To understand organizational structure, we need to integrate the issues of the organization's culture, politics, and stage of growth with its actual organizational reporting structure. Figure 4.1 illustrates the three-dimensional nature of this analysis. We examine each of the three dimensions separately and then integrate the three dimensions with the centralized, decentralized, and matrix types of structure.

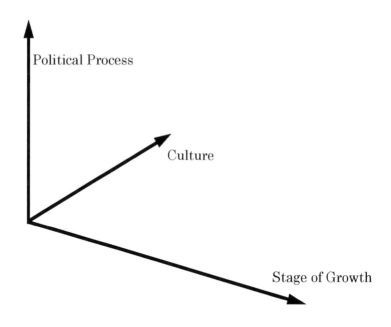

Figure 4.1 Three-dimensional organizational analysis.

The Organization's Culture

The active use of the organizational culture concept by senior managers in organizations is a relatively new phenomenon. Five years ago, the phrase *corporate culture* was rarely heard in health care organizations. Today, it is commonly heard. *Corporate* or *organizational culture* refers to the behavioral characteristics that people within organizations display as they interact with each other and senior management to accomplish their job duties. Some behavioral interactions are positive, some negative. The culture of an organization is the culmination of the behavioral experiences and interactions that members of the organization share in common.

In a large complex health care environment with its many professional and support groups, vastly different views of the organization's culture may coexist. For example, one group may believe that there is a positive culture and that most people are "on board" and working toward a common mission in a cooperative manner. Others may feel that the organization has a dysfunctional culture because of their perception of how they have been treated within the organization and some of the interpersonal problems that they have experienced. This latter group may actually bear organizational "scars" from having needed information withheld, from being the targets of snide comments and innuendoes about their competence, or from other forms of perceived abuse. Still others may behave in condescending ways, especially to "inferiors," using this behavior to maintain their shaky egos by demeaning others.

How people treat and interact with each other in organizations derives from the values of both the organization and the individuals. *Values* are those basic assumptions or beliefs that people and organizations possess about what ideals are worth striving to meet or accomplish. Values are then either reinforced or denied by the actual behaviors of the organization, regardless of what is proclaimed by plaques upon the walls. How is information communicated to staff? Is it aggressively communicated internally or are the employees left to discover major organizational milestones from the local media? What types of memos are sent to staff ? Are these memos direct, paternalistic, nurturing, supportive, etc.? Who is included in the organization's meetings, etc.? Virtually every action in an organization conveys in some way the values that are present. Also, there are subcultures within complex organizations. In a complex health center, there are departments, divisions, units, levels of management, etc. "Each has its own special interests, mental model of how the business works, and quite possibly, its own language (jargon)."[1]

One major study of organizational culture presents seven measures that have high levels of reliability and validity for the dimensions of culture. According to Pliskin et al.[2] these seven measures are as follows:

1. *Innovation and action orientation.* What is the orientation toward progress and change? How well and how quickly does the organization respond to both opportunities and threats in its environment? As an example, the typical bureaucracy would rank low on this while small entrepreneurial organizations would tend to rank much higher. This is similar to what Peters and Waterman[3] characterized as the "Ready, Fire, Aim" attitude.

2. *Risk taking.* Does the organization tend to avoid risk or manage risk? When it looks at decisions in purchasing, investing, hiring, etc., does it focus more on the downside risks or on the potential upside gains?

3. *Integration and lateral interdependence.* What value is placed upon cooperation and communication among subunits in the pursuit of common goals as opposed to the building

and maintenance of fiefdoms? Are open communications encouraged or is information commonly hoarded to gain power? In simplest terms, what value is placed upon teamwork and being a team player?

4. *Top management contact.* Is the manager-subordinate relationship a supportive one? Is there a pervasive concern for employee welfare and growth? Are employees encouraged to speak openly to managers or is the norm to be a "yes person"?

5. *Autonomy in decision making.* Is there a high degree of delegation or is decision authority closely hoarded at higher levels? Are the employees empowered to act on their own to satisfy customers, for example?

6. *Performance orientation.* Are employees under more pressure to perform or to conform? Are results or activities considered more important? Are performance expectations clearly defined? Do the employees feel they are indeed accountable for producing results?

7. *Reward orientation.* Are the employees paid competitive and equitable salaries? Are compensation decisions directly linked to performance? What is the basis for performance appraisals? How are nonmonetary "goodies" allocated?

When considering resistance to the implementation of an information technology system, one cannot explain resistance in terms of the system alone or the people alone. The role of culture—both presumed and actual—must also be considered. Information system designers must be aware of the implications of these cultural issues. One of the first keys is to understand the culture of the total organization and the subunits most involved in the implementation effort.

There is no simple measure of the exact culture in an organization or its subunits. There are simply too many variables involved. However, Table 4.1 presents a scale that can be used to estimate where a given organization stands on the seven measures of culture described above. This can be especially valuable when trying to organize thoughts about the differences between the subunits of an organization.

Whether the total score is 7 or 28, this scale will help you focus your strategies based on the realities of the organization in question.

Orientation to:	Low		High	
1. Action and innovation	1	2	3	4
2. Risk taking	1	2	3	4
3. Cooperation	1	2	3	4
4. Openly supportive management	1	2	3	4
5. Decision-making autonomy	1	2	3	4
6. Clearly defined performance expectations	1	2	3	4
7. Pay for performance	1	2	3	4

Table 4.1. Quick scale to rate an organization's culture.

The Organization's Information Politics

For many people in organizations, *politics* is indeed a dirty word. This is especially true for people with technical backgrounds of various types. First, many associate the word with actual politicians who are often not regarded as one of our higher life forms. More important, politics is squishy! Many people, especially among the technically trained, prefer a world that has (1) well defined variables; (2) logical relationships among these variables; and (3) problems that can be solved, not just coped with.

In more general terms, these people are often more comfortable dealing with concepts or things rather than people. However, organizations are made up of people and inevitably contain complex political relationships.

Davenport et al.[4] conducted a two-year study of information management approaches in more than twenty-five companies. They found that many of the efforts to create information-based organizations or even to implement significant information management initiatives either have failed or are on the way to failure. They contend that failures occur because the companies do not adequately manage the *politics of information*. These failed or failing implementations either tried to apply inappropriate initiatives for their firm's political culture or the political aspects were ignored rather than blended into the initiatives.

Davenport et al. identified five political models in the information arena:

+ technocratic utopianism,
+ anarchy,
+ feudalism,
+ monarchy, and
+ federalism.

Many organizations have one or more of these models present. To manage information and information functions more effectively, the first step is to identify which models exist within the organization, select the most desirable one from an organizational perspective, and then work toward uniformity within the organization. Maintaining multiple models is confusing and consumes scarce resources both inside and outside the information function.

Technocratic Utopianism

Just as the true romanticist believes that love conquers all, the true *technocratic utopian* believes that technology will do the same. The organizational and people issues that are the focus of this book are judged to be irrelevant, inconsequential, and/or "someone else's worry." This model does not focus on the needs of the users; it focuses instead on the activities of the producers, i.e., the technocrats. This is a common model when the core business of the organization is far removed in a knowledge and skills sense from the information technology area. In this type of arena, the technocrats can form a closed society with their own culture, language, and rituals. This separation has been the traditional norm in the health care area.

Until the advent of the microcomputer, information technology was the sole province of the technocrats in many organizations. In fact, these technocrats were often aggressive opponents of the introduction of micros or distributed computing into their organizations, often conducting "guerrilla" warfare to protect their "turf."

Like technologists in many areas—including medicine—utopian information technologists often follow the credo, "If we can, we should." Unfortunately, this is often combined with an exaggerated opinion of what they even "can" do. They tend to love cutting-edge technologies, believing that these will solve many of the existing problems. Their common answer to many complaints about existing systems is, "That will be taken care of in the next release," or "As soon as we get the new server. . ."

The utopians hold two extremely unrealistic beliefs that are often their ultimate downfall:

- ◆ Their tools and technologies are or soon will be the answer to every information problem in the organization.
- ◆ Their failures are not their fault if the organization does not operate in a completely logical and rational manner, like their systems.

These two very unrealistic assumptions are why they are called utopians, believers in a world that never was and never will be.

Anarchy

Anarchy is the absence of an alternative prevailing model. Typically, no one has consciously chosen this state. The organization has drifted into it through the failure of one of the other models or through the failure of the organization to provide a model. Everyone needs information to function. Since there is no unified approach to information in the anarchy model, individuals or subunits collect, accumulate, process, analyze, update, etc., their own information in whatever manner they see as best for them. There were many examples of partial anarchy in the 1980s as individuals learned that they could use microcomputers to do for themselves what unresponsive data processing departments were unwilling or unable to do for them.

The costs of anarchy are obvious: systems that cannot communicate, redundant and inefficient efforts, inaccurate and conflicting data, etc. However, there are two potential positive factors. People do tend to get their individual needs met, and there often is a release of creativity that is not present in more formal systems. However, over any extended period the costs typically far outweigh the benefits.

Feudalism

Information feudalism is a common model that draws its name from the historic model of kings, barons, etc. Ambitious barons attempt to build the power of their individual fiefdoms and jockey for power both with the king and among themselves. In this model, information is the major source of that power. The individual barons decide what, when, and how information will be gathered, processed, stored, and shared. Given the competitive aspect almost inherent in this model, the barons are especially averse to sharing any information that is negative about their fiefdom or its performance. A worse case occurs when they fail to share information that could be helpful to other segments of the organization, not wanting them to look good. This error of omission borders on sabotage, from the perspective of the overall organization. In this model, however, only the king and the immediate royal court care about that overall perspective.

The feudal model is common in companies organized along strong, distinct divisional lines. The strong divisions build their own systems to meet their own needs, both operational and political. In many academic medical centers, there have been attempts to build similar models when the academic departments have had a tradition of high autonomy.

In this feudal model, the head of the organization, the king, can spend large amounts of time and effort attempting to get cooperation among the barons. Issues such as data communication and transfer standards are very hard to achieve because the barons perceive them as threatening their power. In addition, the king may be attempting to make decisions without being able to trust fully the quality of data provided—or not provided—by the barons.

There can be some positive aspects to this model. While the divisions may lose from not fully sharing resources and information with the rest of the organization, the systems that the division does develop should be well tailored to its precise needs. This can be important when the needs of the divisions are quite diverse. A more centralized model often produces compromise systems that please no one. Also, there can be limited collaboration in a feudal model on truly critical issues.

Monarchy

Just as feudalism represents a highly decentralized model, the *monarchy model* describes a highly centralized organization with strong central control. If we think of feudalism as a strong baron and weak king model, the monarchy model is the opposite. In this model, a strong central information function is typically established, often headed by someone with a title such as chief information officer (CIO). This CIO has authority—either solid line or heavy dotted line—over the information activities throughout the organization.

The level of the centralization can vary. At one end of the spectrum, the CIO may set centralized standards such as an organization-wide data dictionary or a list of organization-approved and -supported hardware and software. The actual operations of the information function are still carried out at the subunit level with some degree of autonomy. At the other end, the entire information function is centrally managed with a high degree of conformity throughout the entire organization.

Again, there are pros and cons to this model. Uniformity is achieved along with its benefits in terms of ability to communicate throughout the information and make virtually all information available upon demand to top management. Also, certain economies of scale may be attained through centralized purchasing and licensing agreements and standardized training programs. On the con side, centralized models often meet the needs of diverse units rather poorly, and creativity is not encouraged.

Notice that feudalism and monarchy are essentially antithetical models. It is not uncommon to see an organization using one of these two models make a severe swing to the other model when a major general reorganization occurs. This is particularly true when the reorganization occurs in a time of organizational crisis. Over a period of twenty years, several such swings might occur.

Federalism

Federalism is a relatively recent model that has many desirable features for today's larger organizations. Federalism recognizes that in today's complex organizations various subunits may well have conflicting needs and objectives in their legitimate pursuit of common goals. According to Davenport et al.,

> Federalism most explicitly recognizes the importance of politics, without casting it in pejorative terms. In contrast, technocratic utopianism ignores politics, anarchy is politics run amok, feudalism involves destructive politics, and monarchy attempts to eliminate politics through a strong central authority. Federalism treats politics as a necessary and legitimate activity by which people with different interests work out among themselves a collective purpose and means for achieving it.[4]

Federalism has a number of desirable features. In today's business environment, it is the preferred model for large diverse organization's in most circumstances. Its distinguishing feature is the use of negotiation to bring potentially competing and noncooperating parties together.

> Firms that adopt or evolve into this model typically have strong central leadership and a culture that encourages cooperation and learning. However, it takes tough negotiating and a politically astute information manager to make the federalist model work. Such an information manager needs to have the CEO's support (although not too

much support, or a monarchy emerges) as well as the trust and support of the "lords and barons" who run the divisions. He or she needs to understand the value of information itself as well as of the technology that stores, manipulates, and distributes it. Such skills are not widely distributed throughout organizations, even (or perhaps especially) among IS executives.[4]

Federalism as a concept relies upon a perception of benefits at various levels. The units benefit when their contributions allow a stronger whole that they perceive, in turn, to be of value to them. The whole perceives that it benefits from stronger, not weaker, units. Working from these perceptions, the information-sharing arrangements are then negotiated. The success of a federalist approach depends upon breaking down the traditional levels of distrust between "corporate" and the individual units.

An organization's culture indicates the type of politics that will be prevalent within an organization. Organizations that actively use quality programs to focus on problems from interdisciplinary points of view, empower front-line workers to make decisions, work cross-functionally to improve processes, and remove as much as possible the use of fear as a motivator will gravitate toward less destructive forms of power. It is only when people are stuck in situations and they see constant frustration that politics become more and more prevalent.

Organizational Stages of Growth

Organizations are not static entities. As John W. Gardner wrote, "Like people and plants, organizations have a life cycle. They have a green and supple youth, a time of flourishing strength, and a gnarled old age. . . An organization may go from youth to old age in two or three decades, or it may last for centuries."[5] In the same fashion, the subunits of an organization have life cycles. As Larry Greiner stated in his classic article on organizational growth, "Every organization and its component parts are at different stages of development."[6] Identifying and understanding an organization's stage of growth is critical. The stage of growth often explains some of the organization's concerns, practices, strengths, anxieties, weaknesses, etc. Often, the very form of leadership that is needed and rewarded will vary according to the organization's stage of growth.

Greiner defines five distinguishable phases of organizational development, with each stage ending in a management crisis that typically grows out of the very solution to the preceding crisis. The five stages of organizational growth are:

1. *creativity,* in which the organization is born and fights for survival,
2. *direction,* in which the organization becomes formalized and embarks on a period of sustained growth under directive leadership,
3. *delegation,* in which the organization decentralizes to accommodate the needs of various portions of the organization,
4. *coordination,* in which the organization recentralizes to achieve greater coordination and control, and
5. *collaboration,* in which the organization develops an organizational form tailored to its particular needs and aimed at overcoming the bureaucracy inherent in stage 4.

Greiner refers to the stages as being *evolutionary* and the traumatic passages between stages as being *revolutionary.* While the evolutionary phase of each stage stems from the *dominant management style* used to achieve growth, the revolutionary period is characterized by the *dominant management problem* that must be solved before growth can continue.

Stage 1

Stage 1 is typified by the entrepreneurial start-up situation, whether a small company or small blue sky project team in a larger organization. Stage 1 is often a fight for survival. This is usually the most exciting time in an organization's existence. Circle A in Figure 4.2 depicts the original organization chart for a stage 1 organization—regardless of what the organization might say it is. The spokes indicate the original employees, and show everyone reporting to the hub (which might be more than one person).

The people are committed, often working long hours without any extra compensation. There are two major reasons why these people are so committed:

+ "A place in the sun." For most people, this is the first time they have ever come into direct personal contact with a strong dedicated leader who, by the way, may be one of the worst managers in the Western world. Many people have only worked for job fillers, and this close exposure to dedication and intensity is contagious.

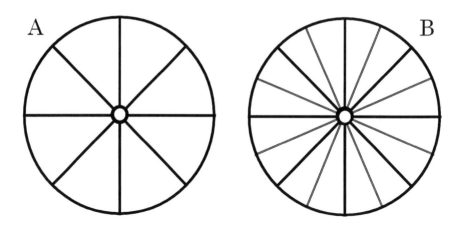

Figure 4.2. Organization chart for a stage 1 organization before and after growth occurs.

♦   All the people in the small organization see the big picture and their places in it. People worry about actually being missed if they are absent for a day; they are not concerned with how many sick days they have left.

This is a stage of high communication and low organization. Communication is almost by osmosis. Everyone knows everything. In fact, confidentiality is almost nonexistent. Figure 4.2 uses wagon wheels as the basic shape rather than asterisks to illustrate just this point. The rim of the wheel indicates that information flows freely, not just through the hub. When systems even exist in stage 1, they are weak. Inventory control consists of someone shouting, "My God, we're out!" However, a critical aspect of stage 1 is that when these crises occur, people do not sit around and point fingers. Instead, everyone, regardless of position, leaps in and helps out. The emphasis in stage 1 is survival, and the organization perceives that the answer to survival is through creativity and growth. In small companies, the answer to every crisis is "sell more," even though they may not know if they are making money on the sales because of the sloppy systems.

The crisis in stage 1 is the crisis in *leadership*. Circle B in Figure 4.2 schematically shows what occurs as the organization grows by adding "spokes" that start to overload the hub. Soon, there are not enough hours in the day for the hub to provide the necessary leadership. In addition, hubs are often not renowned for their willingness or ability to delegate. The hub realizes that if the organization is to survive, "We've got to get organized!"

Stage 2

Stage 2 is a very common stage and one that can last a long time in the absence of high growth. Figure 4.3 shows the stage 2 organizational form. Here we see for the first time the rather standard type of organization chart with the organization typically divided into functional areas and subareas. In a hospital, examples of functional areas are nursing, laundry, billing, information systems, etc.

In this stage, leadership starts to be replaced by administration or direction. Organization, systems, and efficiency are the watchwords of this stage. Now there is a computerized inventory control system that tracks our usages and generates purchase orders when inventory falls to the reorder points. The entire system becomes more formal. We now have "channels of communication," and we start to develop manuals that tell how to do everything. We now know what things cost us, and we focus on improving efficiency and reducing costs.

Motivation and commitment usually fall off in stage 2 compared with the intensity of stage 1. Clouds in the form of intermediate organizational layers start to shield lower level people from the sun. People no longer see the big picture and their places in it. If they attempt to comment or make suggestions on the big picture, they are often told to worry about their own jobs. Work for these people goes from being a quasi-religion to being a "job." In turn, this often leads to the hub complaining about the current employees' lack of

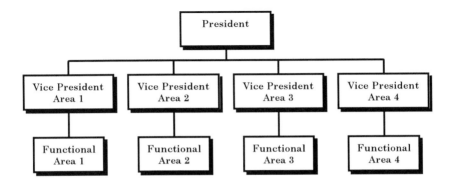

Figure 4.3 Stage 2 organization chart.

dedication and commitment even though this is an understand-able—and even predictable—phenomenon.

There is one potentially distressing aspect that can occur in stage 2, especially in high growth situations. Often as the transition occurs from stages 1 to 2, the top position as shown in Figure 4.3 is taken by the hub. The next level of positions, e.g., the vice presidents, often come from the original or at least the early spokes. Unfortunately, these selections are not made because of the peoples' capabilities to function at high levels in a rapidly growing organization. Rather, they are made because of loyalty and the fact that these early spokes "bled" when there was bleeding to be done. Unfortunately, at some point in stage 2 there is often more bleeding, namely one or more bloodbaths in which some or all of the second-level people have to go. This can happen to the hub, too. This is often one of the sadder times of the organization's existence.

As mentioned earlier, stage 2 can last for a long time. Many departments in larger organizations function at this stage through-out their existence. However, stage 2 can be doomed by certain types of continued organizational growth, namely, growth that brings distinct diversity into the operations of the organization. For example, suppose a health care organization starts to serve two very different markets, such as indigent care and the "silk stocking" market, or starts to function in very different geographic areas with different needs and characteristics. Now the extensive rules and procedures developed within stage 2 can become a hindrance. The voices from these new areas start to cry, "You don't know what it's like to operate here. We need more autonomy." The organization starts to sink under the weight of its centralized procedures.

Stage 3

Stage 3, which Greiner describes as delegation, is probably more widely thought of as decentralization. Figure 4.4 illustrates the divisional structure of a definite stage 3 organization. There is a small "corporate staff" and virtually all activities occur in the various divisions. If the heads of the various divisions are real tigers, this is a stage of explosive growth for many organizations. In stage 2, we had one unit growing; in stage 3, we can have multiple stage 2-type units growing for us. Under good leadership, this stage is so successful because the various divisions can adjust to meet the precise needs of their various markets. Conversely, if the division leaders are weaklings, then stage 3 essentially collapses back to stage 2 as the division leaders do nothing or constantly call home for decisions.

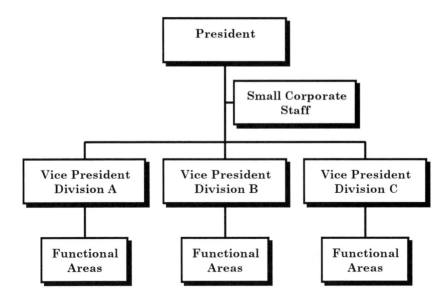

Figure 4.4. Stage 3 organization chart.

As in previous stages, the very success of stage 3 often causes its demise. Almost inevitably in a successful stage 3, the division heads build power and become the strong barons similar to the feudal information model discussed earlier. In fact, that feudal model and stage 3 growth often go together. This strength of the barons starts to make the king nervous, especially if the barons start to flaunt their power. As an example, the corporate staff asks one of the divisions why it made a certain decision. The division response is, "Did we accomplish our goals last year?" When corporate says, "Well, yes you did." The division then tells corporate what it can do with its question, often in impolite terms. This leaves corporate with the uncomfortable feeling that it has responsibility for the overall organizational performance, but that somewhere it has lost the necessary authority. An example of this model at work can be seen at work in an academic medical center in which there are strong department heads and a weak dean.

The term given to this conflict toward the end of stage 3 is *crisis of control*, the control of the central organization over the divisions. Another major complaint made against stage 3 organizations is the "unnecessary" duplication of resources at the divisional level. The argument is often made that many things could be done on a corporate-wide basis much more efficiently. This claim may or may not have merit; however, it often provides a supposed economic basis for moving away from stage 3.

Stage 4

Stage 4 is referred to as a stage of coordination, although a more common term would be *centralization*. The typical tool to achieve this coordination is the buildup of corporate staff. The first thing the members of this expanded staff do is hire their own staffs and then start to write corporate-wide manuals to begin the enforcement of corporate uniformity.

As shown in Figure 4.5, this stages sees the emergence of the *dotted line* on the organization chart. Many of the functions—and especially the staff functions—will now have a dotted line reporting relationship to an executive at corporate. This leaves the formerly autonomous barons in a relatively uncomfortable position. They now have people on their staffs who may have divided loyalties. Moreover, they suspect that some of these people may now feel their career future lies with corporate, which may make their loyalty to corporate the stronger of the two. We know that this organizational form can work, as it is a common one. The price is that the staff members who have two bosses must please both—or at least

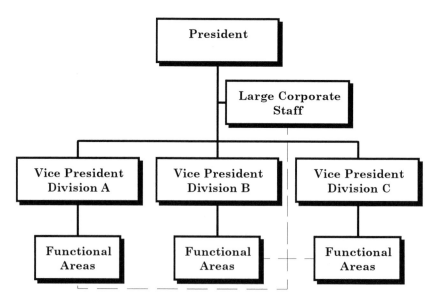

Figure 4.5. Stage 4 organization chart.

displease both equally. This means endless meetings, countless memos, and a continual concern for self-protection. Solutions tend to be compromises rather than being incisive or creative. On the other hand, uniformity across the organization is achieved.

The problem with stage 4 is the organizational overhead it imposes. The costs of running the organization can skyrocket compared with the basic cost of the organizational output. This is referred to as the crisis of red tape. As an example, the United States Navy has more admirals on active duty today than at the height of World War II, despite the fact that today's Navy in total is a small fraction of the earlier size. Left unchecked, stage 4 organizations can grow into enormous bureaucracies. When these organizations meet with a crisis, they often have to form "tiger teams" or "hit squads" or the like to cut through the bureaucracy.

Where the pressures to end stage 3 were primarily internal, the pressures to end stage 4 are typically external. The "market" tells the organization in one way or another that its costs are too high. Something has to be done if the organization is to survive.

Stage 5

Some organizations are able to go on to a stage 5, which Greiner describes in terms of the word *collaboration*. However, stage 5 can be only loosely defined in the sense that some organizations are able to create relatively *unique* organizational forms that meet their particular needs. A classic example of this is Procter and Gamble developing the brand management form of matrix management to meet its particular needs. A general characteristic of these stage 5 organizations is that they expend heavy resources on staff development because these more collaborative forms of organization place heavy demands upon skills such as communications, negotiating, and conflict resolution.

What About the Rest?

What happens to those organizations unable for whatever reasons to make the transformation into a stage 5 model. These organizations typically fall into a pendulum-type pattern, oscillating between stage 3 and stage 4. However, as with a physical pendulum, the oscillation tends to dampen over time. The organization that reverts from stage 4 to stage 3 does not necessarily return to as extreme a decentralization model as it used the first time through the process and likewise again when it reverts back to stage 4. People who are with such an organization over a period of years have this haunting feeling of having seen all this happen before.

Assessing Your Organization

Five scenarios depicting various stages of organizational growth are briefly described below. Pick an overall organization and select the description that best describes that organization. Next, pick another level of the same organization, e.g., a single department or division, and select the best description. Are your choices the same? Why or why not?

- The organization is small and informal. The staff forms a close group. The head knows the names and a modest amount of information about every individual person. There is an esprit de corps among the staff and a feeling that the group can conquer almost any obstacle. There are no layers of administrative or management type staff between the head and the "doers." The people will "roll up their sleeves" and do what has to be done regardless of their positions or titles. The head is very entrepreneurial in gaining money, staff, new ventures, etc. The control systems are loose and unsophisticated. The systems appear to be in a state of continual growth and can be summarized as very flexible. .

- The organization is somewhat centralized and the head and one or two key staff supply virtually all the initiative for instituting modifications to the organizational direction. Time is devoted to establishing policies and procedures, and staff members are required to follow established standards. There is a need to "get organized," which means more structure and the need to plan. There is a greater emphasis on cost reduction than on revenue increase.

- Distinct units or divisions have been created with appointed people responsible for each component. The director's communication with people who actually deliver the service is infrequent and visits to the service site by the director are usually brief. The director spends more time working on new areas rather than working with the day-to-day operations of the department. Budget control is passed downward from the director's office. The people running portions of the department want to be more autonomous and for the director to "loosen the reins."

- The department has become very global and the director feels that there is a need to "tighten the reins." The director requires extensive planning from all key department staff. The department now requires extensive technical support to aid in the department's decision making. A "we/they" attitude between some of the operational people and the administrative and planning people surfaces. It is necessary to establish procedures to review the plans of the operational staff. It is important for people to justify their requests and pans, thus allowing the subunit's goals to be more in alignment with the department's goals.
- A very large department is operated by a series of interdisciplinary groups. The groups are completely accountable for the system they operate. The system is research oriented and encourages innovation. All staff, both professional and support staff, are expected to be self-disciplined in support of the delivery of the best services possible.

Types of Organizational Structures

Whether we read John Naisbitt's *Megatrends* or our daily newspapers, we are constantly told that we are in the "information age."[7] There are statements about how the world is rapidly becoming a global information-based society. Statements and pronouncements about this are found in such diverse sources as magazines, comic strips, television, radio, and the backs of buses. We all know that this is true, but on a day-to-day basis, how do we make the information age become a reality? The concepts of the information age are overwhelming and our resources are limited. What do we do in our health care environments to "move forward"?

As discussed above, organizations of any size usually adopt—knowingly or unknowingly—one of three organizational forms: centralized, decentralized, or matrix.

Centralized

In this model there is normally a central information leader, usually called a chief information officer (CIO), although this person's official title will often vary. All resources that are considered part of the information realm are included under this person's area of responsibility. These areas can include the computing center (data), telecommunications infrastructure (voice and data), television (video), libraries, graphic arts, research facilities, private practice billing functions, and so forth.

Control and responsibility for the informatics function rests with the CIO, who reports to the senior person within the organization. As we look at the stages of organization growth, we see that there are two stages that support the "centralized" system, stage 2 and stage 4. In stage 2, the organization is in a high stage of growth. The senior leader provides the organizational vision and typically maintains high control in the implementation of it. The information technology leader works in conjunction with the organization's leader, and information technology is usually critical to the stage 2 success in today's organizations.

In stage 4, the political environment can be characterized as monarchy and/or technical utopianism. Monarchy occurs because of the stage of growth and the philosophy of the organization's senior leader. Whether technical utopianism occurs depends upon the orientation of the CIO and the staff in the information services department.

Decentralized

Organizations that have a decentralized approach to information systems management say that those with content expertise should be in charge of their subsystem. Several information-based resources that are considered central to the total organization's success are centralized, but most of the information units that are responsible for specific areas remain as independent units. The central office manages the technical infrastructure of the organization and those in the units must be sure that their resources both link to and are integrated into the infrastructure of the system. There is a coordinating and integrating organization structure, usually a council or committee, to ensure parallel goals and directions to fulfill the organizations vision. Most organizations following this model are in organizational growth stage 3.

The political state in this stage of growth could be either feudalism or federalism. In feudalism, the goal of the subunits is to retain information and not readily share it with other members of the organization. Federalism on the other hand has the autonomous subunits sharing information for the good of the whole. Technical utopianism could still prevail in this stage of growth and that philosophy rests with the information systems staff.

Matrix

In the matrix system the organization adopts a combination centralized/decentralized model along with a special unit designed to investigate the concepts, principles, and directions in medical informatics. This unit also works with the end users to develop the new direction and philosophy. The research and development unit creates the "future" while working closely with both end users and the central/decentral unit(s). Once new efforts are ready to be operationalized, they are then handed off to the central/decentral organizations to implement

Organizations that have a true matrix system are generally in organizational growth stage 5, and the political environment is typically characterized as federalism.

We have not included stage 1 as this is such an early stage of an organization's growth that it does not readily fit into today's complex health care environment. It may fit a subunit, but not the total organization. Also while anarchy may seem the prevalent focus in a health care environment today, in reality there is little anarchy.

Conclusion

It is critical to keep these organizational issues in mind while working through the chapters in this section and when trying to put them in practice. The organizational culture, the organization's approach to information management, the organization's stage of growth, and its organizational form all affect the way that information systems can be successfully implemented. Information systems are not implemented in a vacuum. Understanding the organizational milieu is essential. In the next chapters, we will look at practical techniques to use in these various organizational milieus.

Questions

1. During which stage of organizational growth is it easier to implement an integrated information system? Why?
2. What potential advantages might the federalism political model have for clinicians?
3. In which two organizational growth phases will a CIO have a higher probability for success? Why?

4. Name four measures of organizational culture and explain the importance of these measures in understanding an organization's culture.
5. What strategies and tactics might be useful in breaking down technocratic utopianism when it exists in an organization?

References

1. Hodgetts, RM, Luthans, F, Lee, SM. New paradigm organizations: From total quality to learning to world-class. *Organizational Dynamics* 1994;Winter: 5–19.
2. Pliskin, N, Romm, T, Lee, AS, Weber, Y. Presumed versus actual organizational culture: Managerial implications for implementations of information systems. *Computer Journal* 1993;36:143–152.
3. Peters, TJ, Waterman, RH Jr. *In Search of Excellence:Lessons from America's Best-Run Companies.* New York: Harper and Row, 1982.
4. Davenport, TH, Eccles, RG, Prusak, L. Information politics. *Sloan Management Review* 1992; Fall:53–65.
5. Gardner, JW. How to prevent organizational dry rot. *Harper's Magazine* October, 1965;30.
6. Greiner, LE. Evolution and revolution as organizations grow. *Harvard Business Review* 1972:50:(July-August);37–46.
7. Naisbitt, J. *Megatrends: Ten New Directions Transforming Our Lives* New York: Warner Books, 1982.

5
Preparing the Organization for Change

Today's health care organizations are under tremendous stress. Forces such as the current explosions in medical and information technology, the demands of employees for empowerment, financial crises, and demands for major system reform are all forcing today's health care organizations to realize that major change is necessary to be more effective in the future. Many of these organizations affected by significantly changing environmental pressures will have to modify their organizational behaviors and even their structures in major ways.

Critical Skills at Various Management Levels

The need for making major changes starts at the conceptual level. When we view majestic buildings, companies with outstanding profits, or a program so excellent it makes us envious, we need to step back and realize that these outcomes normally did not occur overnight. They started at the conceptual level. Then there was commitment and an understanding of what needed to occur to make that outcome happen. With a new building, someone first needed to decide that a building was needed for a specific purpose. Then the issues of where, when, how, etc., needed to be considered. The time and effort spent well before the ground breaking occurs largely determine the ultimate value of all the activities performed from the ground breaking to the completion of the building.

Years ago, Robert L. Katz[1] stated that there are three basic types of skills that a person must have in order to be a good manager: conceptual, human, and technical skills. The *conceptual skills* are used to see the enterprise as a whole, including the relationships of all the various parts to the whole and to each other. The conceptual skills also extend to visualizing the relationship of the overall organization to the industry, the community, and to all the political, social, and economic forces at work. The *human skills* are used to build teams that work together and interact effectively with other levels and areas of the organization. The *technical skills* are used to directly supervise specific operational activities, particularly those involving detailed methods, processes, procedures, or techniques.

To survive and to achieve future success, organizations must have these three components, whether they are a four-person consulting business, an 800-person manufacturing business, or a 4,000-person hospital. Figure 5.1 graphically depicts Katz's basic concepts of the levels of managerial concern within organizations. Figure 5.2 shows the most critical skills at each of these three levels. Like all models, this one is a simplification of reality, as it shows three distinct levels to represent what, in fact, is a continuum of both the primary concerns and the critical skills.

At the base level of an organization, the technical skills are the most critical ones because the primary concern at that level is the production of the goods and services that justify the organization's existence. In a health care environment, these products and services are treatments for patients, examinations and tests such as mammograms and magnetic resonance imaging (MRIs), the education of students or staff, and so forth.

Figure 5.1 shows that the management of the organization and its people is the primary concern in the middle range of the organization. Therefore, the human skills are the most critical as shown in Figure 5.2. Hospitals and health organizations have implemented many different types of internal people-focused programs such as Continuous Quality Improvement. Other examples are "guest

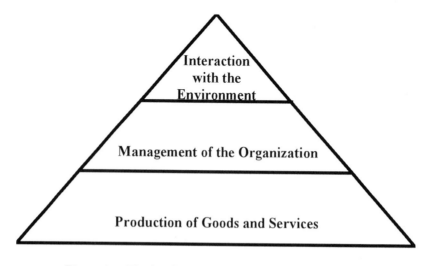

Figure 5.1. The levels of primary management concern.

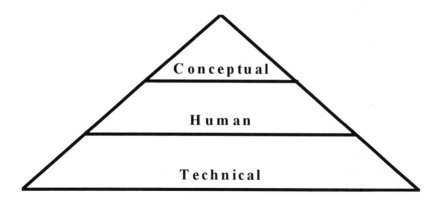

Figure 5.2. Critical management skills for each level of primary concern.

relations" or year-of-the-customer programs to teach to the staff the skills for interacting with the hospitals' publics. These people issues are at the heart of management process.

Figure 5.1 shows that the interaction with the environment is the primary management concern at the upper levels of the organization. Now, the conceptual skills are the most critical as shown in Figure 5.2. What business are we in? What business should we be in five years from now?

When talking about the conceptual level, an often used classical example is the manufacture of buggy whips. When the automobile industry was in its infancy, there were many companies making buggy whips. Many of these companies merely laughed at the noisy, unreliable new contraptions called automobiles and continued their long-run plans for making buggy whips. Of course, the outcome was highly predictable for those companies that did not adapt. Fifteen years ago, employees of a major x-ray film manufacturer laughed when we mentioned that digital imaging would eventually have a significant impact on their markets. They immediately started talking about what their technology could do compared with the mediocre quality of the digital imaging of that era. None of them seemed to appreciate that they were comparing the attributes and qualities of a relatively mature technology to those of a technology in its infancy that had enormous potential. We wonder how many of those people still have their jobs.

An example of a successful redefinition of a company's products and services is the Procter and Gamble Company. As the corporate folklore goes, Procter and Gamble created Ivory soap through a serendipitous mistake. During the normal manufacturing process someone allowed the blending machine to run too long one day, which introduced a great deal of air into the product. Because of this accidental aeration, the resulting bars of soap floated. This "problem" quickly turned into a bonanza, and Ivory soap became the keystone product in the growth of Procter and Gamble into a major international corporation. Today, the Procter and Gamble Company continues to understand its environment and to conceptually plan ahead.

Throughout the above discussion, we have talked about the critical skills at each general level of the organization. In reality, the three major skills are all important at all levels of the organization. The question is the balance, as illustrated schematically in Figure 5.3. The sizes of the letters C for Conceptual, H for Human, and T for Technical at each level give an indication of their relative importance. The largest letter at each level denotes the skill we previously identified as the critical one.

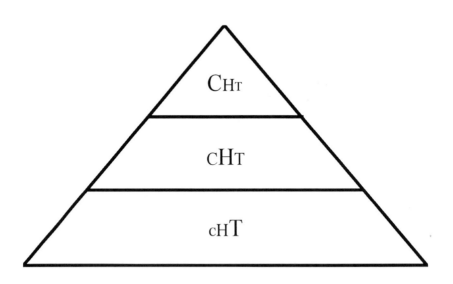

Figure 5.3. Relative importance of the three critical skills at the three levels of management.

Critical Issues for Change

Ensuring successful changes requires that we make appropriate use of all three of the critical management skills discussed above. In addition, we must address the following seven crucial areas:

1. making proactive vs. reactive change,
2. understanding the critical global and local issues,
3. creating a vision for change,
4. identifying the key change leader characteristics,
5. gaining commitment from the organizational leadership,
6. defining the end-user needs, and
7. appreciating organizational stress.

Making Proactive vs. Reactive Changes

In the late 1940s, W. Edwards Deming was preaching the quality system that he had developed during the 1930s. However, the United States was embarking on the greatest economic boom in the history of the world, producing a flood of goods desired all over the war-torn world. Not only were Deming's pleas for his quality system rejected, he was castigated as someone who did not understand the philosophy and directions of business. The old joke is that a person is an expert only when more than 50 miles away from home. Deming had to be halfway around the world. The Japanese in the postwar years were desperate to determine their future strategies and directions. Using Deming's methods, the Japanese improved their production quality tremendously within a decade and started to capture various markets around the world.

The initial Japanese acceptance of Deming's message can probably be thought of as reactive, a response to the terrible quality image that Japanese products had at the time. However, in his conferences with senior leaders of Japanese companies, Deming convinced them that quality was the way to the future. In a very proactive manner, the Japanese listened to Deming. They did not merely try to catch up with world standards in quality, they created new world class standards for quality, leaving the rest of the world to scramble frantically in pursuit.

Deming was a fervent voice for proactive change, preaching the message of quality whether it was popular or not. He looked at the long-term consequences of quality in a very positive and proactive way. The pursuit of quality has become a major effort in the world today, especially in the United States. This pursuit began in manufacturing and has moved into the service industries, including the health care area. We cannot go into many health care institutions today without immediately hearing about their Total Quality Management or Continuous Quality Improvement programs.

In *Workplace 2000*, Joseph Boyett and Henry Conn[2] acknowledge the high need for quality but predict that those who adopt mechanistic approaches to improving quality will find people focusing on filling out forms rather than improving quality. This is basically what happened to management by objectives (MBO), which many organizations tried in the 1970s and early 1980s. Most organizations *reactively* adopted the processes and rituals rather than *proactively* adopting the philosophies and intent. Many of these same organizations are still trying one packaged fad program after another, not realizing—or perhaps not wanting to admit—where their real problem lies. Boyett and Conn indicate that quality is critical to success, but unless the philosophy of quality is built into the total system, it will become one more set of organizational rituals.

Organizational leaders preparing for change must first be aware of why they are engaging in the change. Do they truly wish to make proactive long-range future decisions or do they just want not to be "left out" of the latest organizational fad? How do you know if you are behaving proactively or reactively? Let's look at some examples of the proactive versus reactive questions that organizations ask. Table 5.1 provides some examples of the differences in approach that proactive and reactive leaders would take in asking questions or addressing problems and issues.

In the changing health care environment in which we live, it is important for an institution to remain as proactive as possible. One way to do this is to identify the key or core values and to focus efforts around those key core values. Organizations do not select their key or core values by accident. They select them with a defined strategy and a measurable action plan. Some of the organizational values commonly mentioned are listed in Table 5.2 along with space for you to customize the chart. As it is important for you to assess which are the top values within your organization, we suggest that you use Table 5.2 to record your perceptions of how your organization—both the total organization and your area—specifically ranks these values. Where does your organization stand on each of the values listed? What values are critical in your organization that are not listed?

Proactive Questions	Reactive Questions
1. What type of health care will be needed by our community during the next five years?	1. We are only filling 60% of our beds. We must fill beds or we will lose money. What should we do?
2. What are our strengths in the health care system to address these community health care problems?	2. How can we stop losing market share to hospitals A, B, and C. Some of the least productive hospitals are effectively advertising for services that we know we perform better.
3. What is our strategic vision that incorporates the community needs and our strengths to address those issues? If there are some areas that others do better, we shall partner with them in order to have a comprehensive health care system that we act as a player in, but are not the major player.	3. How can we maintain our position of prestige in this industry unless we compete head-on with hospitals A, B, and C?
4. What information system will best serve the needs of our patients?	4. What information system is the most cost-effective now?
5. Who are the best people to help us decide what system to select?	5. We must control the selection process so we can move fast.

Table 5.1. Comparison of proactive and reactive approaches.

Although all of the values shown in Table 5.2 are positive, no organization can adhere to all of them equally. Most experts suggest selecting one *driving value* from the list and four *facilitating values* in order to keep the organizational priorities sharp. An example of this approach for a particular organization is shown in Table 5.3.

What do you consider to be your organization's Top Driving Value and Four Facilitating Values? If it does not seem to have any, what do you think they should be for the overall organization? For your subunit? Table 5.4 provides the structure for you to answer these questions for your organization or subunit.

Value	Low		Medium		High
Teamwork/Collaboration	❑	❑	❑	❑	❑
Empowerment/Involvement	❑	❑	❑	❑	❑
Innovation	❑	❑	❑	❑	❑
Quality	❑	❑	❑	❑	❑
Sense of Urgency	❑	❑	❑	❑	❑
Risk Taking	❑	❑	❑	❑	❑
Customer Service	❑	❑	❑	❑	❑
Concern for People	❑	❑	❑	❑	❑
Meeting Customer Needs	❑	❑	❑	❑	❑
Maximizing Resources	❑	❑	❑	❑	❑
Cost Consciousness	❑	❑	❑	❑	❑
Continuous Improvement	❑	❑	❑	❑	❑
Trust	❑	❑	❑	❑	❑
_____	❑	❑	❑	❑	❑
_____	❑	❑	❑	❑	❑
_____	❑	❑	❑	❑	❑

Table 5.2. Some alternative organizational core or key values.

We have been primarily addressing the total organization. As we look at the information systems area, we see the same types of things happening on a smaller scale—the proactive versus the reactive changes for information management. Some of the proactive reasons for changing an information system might include:

Top Driving Value:	Meeting Customer Needs
Four Facilitating Values:	1. Teamwork/Collaboration
	2. Concern for People
	3. Sense of Urgency
	4. Maximizing Use of Resources

Table 5.3. Sample set of key and facilitating values.

Top Driving Value:	?
Four Facilitating Values:	1.
	2.
	3.
	4.

Table 5.4. Structure for recording organizational or subunit values.

- our paper systems are fire hazards that really don't meet our information needs and should be modified or eliminated
- the system we have met our needs when we implemented it but now it simply does not enhance the quality of our patient care.

Some of the reactive reasons might include:

- everyone else has one and we should too
- we are going to get clobbered in our accreditation review next year unless we . . . !

To summarize in sports terms, proactive changes are *offensive* changes, that is, moves that support or advance the organizational vision. Using a medical analogy, they are aimed at preventing or curing the *disease*. *Defensive* changes are those that occur for reactive reasons, typically aimed at merely alleviating the *symptoms* of the moment.

Understanding the Critical Global and Local Issues

Change made simply for the sake of change is ineffective as well as being irresponsible management. We must critique potential changes within the context of the total organization and its vision and goals. There are numerous irresponsible contexts in which changes are made. One example is panic in response to power. Someone in power loudly complains, rightly or wrongly, "Our billing system is not worth a damn!" In a panicked reaction, the first available system is seized upon. Another example is changes that are motivated by empire building or résumé building, making hardware or software selections for their résumé value.

Change that is both needed and planned is important to the total institution. Two analyses are necessary to understand what is needed: (1) a full assessment of the global issues, including environment and direction, and (2) a full assessment of the local needs.

Global Issues

There are a number of ways to assess the global issues, and the following are examples of key strategies that organizations have used in the past:

- Seeking out contacts with key leaders in the field to determine their opinions and/or research with regard to current and possible future considerations.
- Identifying the trends through both the literature and key trend documents that may not be officially indexed in the literature. In the general literature, services such as the Popcorn Report discuss general trends for marketing. In the health care industry, there are a number of organizations that offer their opinions of the trends. One such organization is the Program on Information Resources Policy of the Center for Information Policy Research at Harvard University.

- ◆ Benchmarking to determine what leading edge organizations in the field are doing and how they do it. This can be done through surveys, interviews, and site visits.

Interviews and surveys can be powerful tools in obtaining global types of information. An interview, whether over the telephone or in person, can provide a tremendous amount of information. John Naisbitt's *Megatrends*[3] comments about "high tech/high touch" are never more apparent than in the information technology area. Many people will spend hours talking to and helping complete strangers on computer issues, whether technical or people issues.

A well-constructed survey can also gather much valuable information to assist future decisions. Surveys need to have two major characteristics; the survey questions need to be clear, and the entire survey must require only a reasonable amount of effort on the part of the respondents. The survey should be tested first on several people who occupy roles similar to those being sampled to determine if:

- ◆ the survey will actually produce the kind of information that will be helpful and
- ◆ the survey can be answered with reasonable effort.

As a personal example, we have started to answer many surveys only to find that completing them took too long or the poor construction of the survey made it too frustrating to answer the questions easily. In either case, the surveys ended up in the trash, and our opinion of the sender went down accordingly. Proper testing is essential.

Local Issues and Needs

If you were graded on your answers to the questions listed below, would you pass or fail? How well do you really know your organization?

1. Would you call your overall organization a fairly open organization or a fairly hierarchical organization? Why?
2. In your organization, in what order do you see the following behaviors being rewarded?

- ◆ bringing "secret" information or gossip to bosses
- ◆ performing well in terms of results
- ◆ being "yes people" to those in power

- making decisions and taking risks
- being a rigid rule follower
- being a team player
- presenting a good "image"

3. How would you briefly describe the power structure within your organization?
4. What is the balance of power between the people/roles such as presidents, vice presidents, hospital administrators, department chairmen, deans, chiefs of service, etc.?
5. Whose "stars" are rising in your organization? Why?
6. Whose "stars" are falling in your organization? Why?
7. What seemingly negative behaviors are widely tolerated in your organization? Why?
8. What behaviors are definitely not tolerated in your organization? Why?
9. Would you describe your organization as relatively stable or are there definite cultural changes occurring? If yes to the latter, what are they?
10. Is there a norm of peer support within your organization?
11. Is there a norm of supervisory support within your organization?
12. What is the general level of pressure and stress within your organization? If it is high, what is causing it?

Anyone wishing to make changes within an organization with minimum levels of trauma must first understand that organization's milieu. The questions above cover a wide range of issues involving the organization's power bases, structures, reward systems, and so forth. Understanding these issues is a key to developing appropriate strategies at the appropriate times and for involving the key players within the organization. If you find yourself unable to comfortably answer the above questions for an organization in which you have spent over a year, this is a definite indicator that you have an underdeveloped set of organizational antennae. If you do not have the time or desire to change this, you may well need expert outside help to assist in these organizational analyses.

Change leaders can get caught by changes in organizational style and/or the power structure. For example, a major information systems project was started in one organization during the tenure of a particular CEO. Halfway through the project, the organization changed CEOs. The new CEO did not believe in the system and direction that was created under the previous CEO. Although large amounts of time and money had been expended, support for the system dwindled with the new administration indicating to many previous supporters that the system was not worth supporting. Although the project leader had ensured that all the "power bases" were included under the previous regime, the change in top leadership made much of this effort useless. Ultimately, this major system was terminated prior to full implementation, even though the system was respected and deemed important by the end users who had been exposed to it.

As another example, a hospital in a state of change called in an outside consultant who brought together a significant number of the top echelon of the hospital. The consultant asked all members of the middle and upper level management to complete a survey that would identify the style of organization and the organizational issues that we are discussing in this chapter. The consultant promised anonymity to all those who completed the survey, but did request the participants' names to ensure that problems in different subunits could be properly identified to aid in developing appropriate organizational development strategies. Almost 100 percent of the people completed their surveys; however, only 50 percent of the people clearly identified themselves and their areas. The consultant, being a bit perplexed, decided to analyze the data in two groups. The first group included all the people who clearly identified their name and department. The second group included those who completed the survey but did not identify their name or location. The actual compiled results from both groups were virtually identical. However, it was obvious that the latter group did not feel empowered and appeared to feel too threatened to provide any personal data. The consultant returned the individual surveys in sealed envelopes to those who had given their names. During a general feedback session, the unidentified surveys had been left lying on a table as the consultant had no way to identify their owners. After a coffee break, all these unidentified surveys had mysteriously disappeared. In this hospital, there was no trust in the system. This organization was definitely in a state of severe anxiety with many middle and some upper level managers mistrusting the organizational hierarchy. If you were making change in this particular organization, your first step would have to be to address these trust issues directly.

Creating a Vision for Change

Vision—what is it and where do you get it? Do you concentrate on not making buggy whips and become obsessive about that? Do you listen to the rosy promises that vendors whisper in your ear? How do you decide? Where do you begin?

In a personal conversation years ago, Russell Ackoff, one of the great minds in decision making and operations research, observed that we can envision the future; we simply cannot plan for it in great details. He went on to say that everything an organization needs to determine future direction is known today (although we may not know it, of course, if we hide our heads in the sand like a threatened ostrich). While Ackoff's assertion may sound a bit odd, let's look at several recent information technology items that have appeared in print.

> Dun & Bradstreet Software asked many users of mainframe computers what their intentions were regarding mainframe applications through 1995. Result: Only 47% said they intended to buy mainframe applications (as opposed to doing nothing or buying applications based on other classes of computing equipment). Buying software is a big indicator of the attitude people and companies have about the value of hardware. With fewer than half of the companies that use mainframes planning to buy software to run on them, it seems clear that the popularity of these big ugly things has cooled dramatically. Maybe my prediction that the last mainframe will be unplugged on March 15, 1995, isn't quite so nutty after all . . .[4]

> Anthem, a managed care company that services 55 million people, and Paradigm Management, Inc. created a knowledge base using object-oriented programming and relational databases. "We've seen tremendous power and productivity through this teaming of object-oriented and relational technologies. We can develop new types of systems and develop them much more quickly."[5]

> Studies have shown that nurses spend 30 to 40 percent of their time recording information by hand on patient's charts. That, combined with more complex patient acuity and a shortage of nurses, places more demands on nurses' time, clearly demonstrating the need for an efficient system to record the massive amounts of information generated in the nursing setting. The solution is clinical information systems, that is, bedside computers that gather information directly from monitors, other bedside devices, and automated systems within the hospital. Clinical information systems, more than any other development, will change the future of nursing in the next five years. By allowing the nurses to spend less time documenting patient care and

more time administering it, clinical information systems will bring nursing into the 21st century.[6]

System managers are increasingly partnering with end users and business heads. As more organizations move away from traditional computing models, they're discovering that organizational changes are a necessary and integral part of the client/server landscape. End users are playing an increasing role in the management of their data and applications, while IS departments are becoming more involved with the business.[7]

These four excerpts are examples of the types of inputs that informatics leaders require to begin to envision some of the ways that information technology will be able to lead and support the implementation of their parent organizations' visions and missions. We all know that listening to four gurus may produce at least five opinions. In the end, we all have to make our own judgments as to which part of the known information—to use Ackoff's concept—will be most relevant to our case.

The keys to successful creation of a vision are

+ visionary leadership possessing a "can do" attitude,
+ knowledge and understanding of the needs of the major stakeholders, and
+ knowledge and understanding of the organizational milieu, including both the opportunities and the constraints.

These three provide the foundation that enables the creation of a meaningful vision. Once the vision is created, this foundation will also allow the vision statement to be translated strategically into statements of the "we want to be capable of" type. Creating a "capable of" statement is the step that translates the vision into a workable and understandable action-oriented goal. Many people might read the vision statement and say, "That sounds great." Unfortunately, they then return to their regular work, and the vision gathers dust on the shelf. In many ways, a vision is so big that it is somewhat like an elephant. First, the elephant is so big that even people with normal sight can examine it and draw very different conclusions. Second, it is difficult to decide how to "eat" that elephant. Often, there is endless debate about the process; then everyone agrees that it is indeed a beautiful creature but simply too big to eat. The "capable of" statement is action-oriented and helps people dissect an elephant, making the vision more manageable.

As an example of the concepts described above, a *vision statement* might be, "The organization will have a fully integrated information system." One of the many supporting *capable-of statements* might be, "The system will be capable of electronically accessing selected full-text library journal resources from the patient floor." This example clearly shows how "capable of" statements got their name.

In some health care organizations today, there is a continuous battle for leadership and control. In some organizations, the senior leader acts with inputs from only a few hand-picked people. In some other organizations, the corporate culture acknowledges that the challenges of today's health care environment are too great for just a few senior leaders to cope with by themselves. Those developing the information systems to support health care organization must be aware of these issues. In 1958, Robert Tannenbaum and Warren Schmidt[8] published their classic article on selecting a leadership pattern. The article presented an "ask to sell" continuum. Figure 5.4 is an adaptation of their continuum to the health environment.

The more contemporary approach to managing the complexity of the health care situation is to be somewhere in the center or to the right of center of the model. However, if the information systems person is functioning in an environment where the decisions are made on the far left side, then the information system planning needs to first acknowledge this environment and then needs to gather vision ideas from those who are on the right side of the model.

With this analysis completed, it is then necessary to approach the key power brokers within the organization, share the vision (perhaps in draft form) with them, encourage each person to become involved and make inputs, and build ownership in the vision.

If the "capable of" statements seem to be "fuzzy," then it is critical for the person creating the vision statements to remove as much of this fuzziness as possible. When the concept of integrated information (IAIMS) was first presented at the University of Cincinnati Medical Center, it was clear that a few people understood and agreed with what was being said, but there were many "glassy" stares. At that point, the IAIMS leader created a scenario about an imaginary patient, Mary Smith, who became ill at 2 a.m.[9] Each clinical department was then asked what types of information and communication items they would need in order to effectively treat Mary Smith's problems. Poor Mary had many varied problems, of course, depending upon the group being addressed. If it was the Department of Psychiatry, Mary had major psychiatric problems, and the issues of confidentiality received considerable attention. If Mary was a post-op surgical patient, the Department of Surgery would express her complications in a very clear and distinct manner. If the physicians were from Internal Medicine, Mary had many

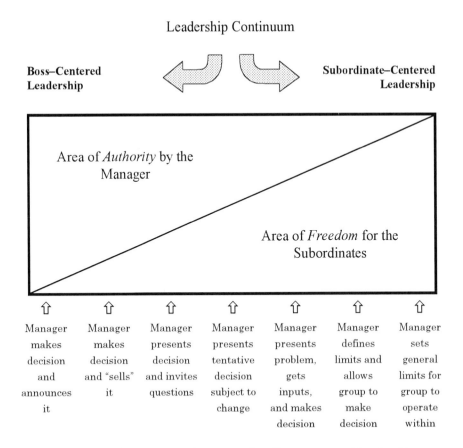

Figure 5.4. Boss-centered versus subordinate-centered leadership.

problems that would pertain to the various specialties within Internal Medicine.

The key IAIMS developers at the University of Cincinnati then took the various visions created about Mary Smith and amalgamated them into a strategic vision of clinical information needs. Once a strategic vision was developed, the "capable of" statements for the system were developed in very clear terms that the systems people could understand. Using this process, the entire vision was created by the clinicians who would be empowered in the long run to use the system on a day-by-day basis.

Identifying the Key Change Leader Concerns

Change leaders who have to function at the "bleeding edge" are not always successful. Always remember, John the Baptist, a change leader proclaiming one of history's largest changes, lost his head! We personally know health care informatics change leaders who have assumed their roles to the blare of trumpets, only to exit in an amazingly short time carried on their shields. To be successful, the informatics change leader must understand and constantly monitor four key concerns:

- point-person role,
- knowledge and commitment,
- formal and informal power, and
- rapid shifts in focus.

In the following discussion, notice that some of these key concerns may involve issues that need to be resolved before the change leader assumes the role. If these issues cannot be resolved to the change leader's satisfaction, assuming the responsibilities is probably a big mistake.

Point-Person Role

The change leader is the "point" person for the change that happens, and may well become a "symbol" of this change to those unhappy with it. This is a variation on the old "shoot the messenger" phenomenon. Stresses within the organization or the environment that do not directly involve the particular change will still often have an impact on the change leader. Suppose an organization is moving from the "big iron" mainframe-type information systems approach to a more decentralized approach. If the IS staff members feel that they may not have the skills for this new direction and perhaps feel that their future or even their jobs are threatened, they will probably resist the change vigorously. In one organization with more than 100 people in the IS department, volunteers were sought to assist in exploring the new direction for that institution. One person chose to go with the new group. As early small successes started to occur, many of the people within that IS department clearly realized that they did not have the appropriate skills for the future. Rather than upgrading their skills, they spent considerable time and energy resisting the new system and the efforts of the change leader in order to try and stop the system. Eventually the transition was made, but unfortunately the negativity toward the change leader "who had caused all the problems" lingered on.

Knowledge and Commitment

The change leader must be both knowledgeable and committed. Knowledgeable means an understanding of not only the organizational issues but also of the technology and the concept of systems. The person must be respected for his or her particular knowledge and must be firmly committed to the project. Any significant project will inevitably have its moments of euphoria and its moments of despair. A deep commitment—coupled with competence and confidence—is essential for weathering these lows.

Formal and Informal Power

The change leader must have the necessary formal and informal power within the organization to lead the change. The person could have formal organizational power, such as being the CIO, but without personal respect within the organization he or she will not be successful. On the other hand, someone may have high informal power within the organization but without formal power be blocked by a minority of the organization that does not accept that informal power. The change leader must be the authorized or legitimate organizational leader. It is critical that the organization sanction only one person to lead the effort and support that person through the highs and lows of the change process. If "competing" formal leaders are created by the organization, massive resources that could be dedicated to the change process will be wasted in "turf" battles.

Rapid Shifts in Focus

The role of change leader typically requires good skills in the technical, human, and conceptual areas, as discussed earlier. More important, the change leader has to be able to constantly and rapidly shift between these skill areas on any given day. This kind of mental flexibility is critical. While successful change leaders must certainly have the ability to plan and organize well, they must also have the mental flexibility to deal with interruptions, changes in plans, and changes in the area and level of focus.

Organizational Leadership Commitment

Think about a plate of ham and eggs. The chicken is involved, but the pig is committed! The organizational leadership—CEO, president, vice presidents, deans, department chairs, etc.—must be *committed* to supporting the change process, not merely involved. They must ensure that there is broad and constant support for the process and the resulting projects. They must also "stay" with the change process in the sense of ensuring that all their decisions and actions are consistent with the values of the change process. The way for top leadership to kill a change process is for them to establish a vision, send some person or group off to implement that vision, and then proceed to make decisions not in accord with that vision.

It is critical that top management continuously integrates information planning into the overall organizational planning process rather than treating information issues as occasional problems to be solved on a crisis basis. Since health care organizations are so complex and constantly changing, the top organizational leaders are typically involved in the decision to implement major new technology systems. They then normally charge the person managing this effort with completing the implementation. At this point, top management gallops off to deal with other problems, feeling that this particular area has been handled. The information systems people then proceed to build the system that was approved for the organization. Unfortunately, major systems are not implemented overnight. By the time of actual implementation, the system that was envisioned as needed one or two years ago may not be the system that is needed today. When the new system does not meet the current needs of the organization, the day-to-day operational processes and procedures of the organization cannot meet the new needs, but are anchored to the old ways. We leave you to speculate on who takes the blame.

End-User Needs

The end users are key stakeholders in the implementation of any health informatics system. There are five key areas of concern involving these customers for the information system:

1.   The end users must know and comprehend what the system will be realistically capable of doing. In the Mary Smith scenario mentioned earlier, the end users helped create the scenario for the information needs that they had with regard

to Mary Smith. The role of the information managers and leaders is to effectively manage the end-user expectations because the expectations will always be greater than the capabilities of the technology, the software, and the people who can deliver the end products.

2.   The end users must be included in the communications and information regarding changes that are being considered and/or developed.

3.   The end users must believe that key people are committed to the success of the system. In one organization, the department head decide that he would develop a "tiger team" made up of several people from his group plus several people from the information systems group. The team met over a two-month period and, using a very iterative process, developed a system that was accepted immediately. The system worked because the hand-picked user representatives brought high content knowledge to the project *and* constantly discussed progress and needs with their other colleagues. That system is still in use today and continues to be enhanced.

4.   The gatekeepers and opinion leaders must support the system and push or pull through various times of success or failure. The gatekeepers and opinion leaders need not be the formal organizational leadership.

5.   End users must "see and know" the results of their inputs as rapidly as possible. This is true whether it is helping the residency recruitment program, creating a discharge summary statement, clearly identifying all the drugs that a patient is taking, or identifying past medical problems. It is important that changes be seen immediately and not in three to five years after end-user participation in the process.

Stress

When people begin to feel increases in their levels of stress, their excitement for the future may lead to panic, which is a factor in the "stuck" personality described by Rosabeth Moss Kanter.[10] Security in a position allows excitement; insecurity fosters panic. The health care industry is in a very stressful time. The work has always involved a lot of stress. However, with today's political pressures for significant changes in many health care systems, whole new kinds of stress involving job and income security have been added to the mix.

As the stresses become more pronounced, many of the people become engaged in negative behavior. Kanter identifies those people who are "stuck" in an organization as major creators of problems. They engage in gossip, back-stabbing, and outright lack of concern for their jobs and their future. Many of the negative stress comments mentioned in Chapter 2 are heard daily from the more vocal people. Others express their fears and discontent in more silent ways. The challenge to the change leader is to be constantly alert to the symptoms and impacts of stress.

Organizational Readiness for Change

Some organizations seem to handle change comfortably; others resist change ferociously. For example, Warren Bennis once commented to us, "Introducing change in a university is roughly akin to introducing change in a cemetery!" According to George Bennett, CEO of the Symmetrix consulting company, "Some places, we've gone in with our best people and broken our picks. That's a waste of our resources and those of our clients."[11] If you are asked to lead a significant change effort in an organization with a highly resistant culture, you may rapidly begin to feel like a modern Sisyphus. Table 5.5 contains a readiness "quiz" derived from the work of Dr. Andrea Sodana of Symmetrix.[11] The overall score on this quiz will give you a measure of the likely difficulty in introducing change into your organization.

In scoring the quiz, assign three points if you rate your organization highly on this dimension ("We do this well."). Assign two points for a medium rating ("We need to improve on this."). Assign one point for a low rating ("We do this poorly or not at all."). Get inputs from others to supplement or validate your own perspectives and opinions.

Category	Score
Sponsorship The sponsor of change is not necessarily its day-to-day leader; he or she is the visionary, chief cheerleader, and bill payer— the person with the power to help the team change when it meets resistance. Give three points—change will be easier—if sponsorship comes at a senior level; for example, CEO, COO, or the head of an autonomous business unit. Weakest sponsors: midlevel executives or staff officers.	☐
Leadership This means the day-to-day leadership—the people who call the meetings, set the goals, work till midnight. Successful change is more likely if leadership is high level, has "ownership" (that is, direct responsibility for what's to be changed) and has clear business results in mind. Low-level leadership, or leadership that is not well connected throughout the organization (across departments) or that comes from the staff, is less likely to succeed and should be scored low.	☐
Motivation High points for a strong sense of urgency from senior management, which is shared by the rest of the company, and for a corporate culture that already emphasizes continuous improvement. Negative: tradition-bound managers and workers, many of whom have been in their jobs for more than 15 years; a conservative culture that discourages risk taking.	☐
Direction Does senior management strongly believe that the future should look different from the present? How clear is management's picture of the future? Can management mobilize all relevant parties—employees, the board, customers, etc.—for action? High points for positive answers to those questions. If senior management thinks only minor change is needed, the likely outcome is no change at all; score yourself low.	☐

Measurements Or in consultant-speak, "metrics." Three points if you already use performance measures of the sort encouraged by total quality management (defect rates, time to market, etc.) and if these express the economics of the business. Two points if some measures exist but compensation and reward systems do not explicitly reinforce them. If you don't have measures in place or don't know what we are talking about, one point.	☐
Organizational Context How does the change effort connect to other major goings-on in the organization? (For example: Does it fit with strategic actions such as acquisitions or new product lines?) Trouble lies ahead for a change effort that is isolated or if there are multiple change efforts whose relationships are not linked strategically.	☐
Processes/Functions Major changes almost invariably require redesigning business processes that cut across functions such as purchasing, accounts payable, or marketing. If functional executives are rigidly turf conscious, change will be difficult. Give yourself more points the more willing they—and the organization as a whole—are to change critical processes and sacrifice perks or power for the good of the group.	☐
Competitor Benchmarking Whether you are a leader in your industry or a laggard, give yourself points for a continuing program that objectively compares your company's performance with that of competitors and systematically examines changes in your market. Give yourself one point if knowledge of competitors' abilities is primarily anecdotal—what salesman say at the bar.	☐
Customer Focus The more everyone in the company is imbued with knowledge of customers, the more likely that the organization can agree to change to serve them better. Three points if everyone in the work force knows who his or her customers are, knows their needs, and has had direct contact with them. Take away points if that knowledge is confined to pockets of the organization (sales and marketing, senior executives).	☐

Rewards Change is easier if managers and employees are rewarded for taking risks, being innovative, and looking for new solutions. Team-based rewards are better than rewards based solely upon individual achievement. Reduce points if your company, like most, rewards continuity over change. If managers become heroes for making budget, they won't take risks even if you say you want them to. Also: If employees believe failure will be punished, reduce points.	☐
Organizational Structure The best situation is a flexible organization with little churn—that is, reorganizations are rare and well received. Score yourself lower if you have a rigid structure that has been unchanged for more than five years or has undergone frequent reorganization with little success; that may signal a cynical company structure that fights change by waiting it out.	☐
Communication A company will adapt to change most readily if it has many means of two-way communication that reach all levels of the organization and that all employees use and understand. If communications media are few, often trashed unread and almost exclusively one-way and top-down, change will be more difficult.	☐
Organizational Hierarchy The fewer levels of hierarchy and the fewer employee grade levels, the more likely an effort to change will succeed. A thick impasto of middle management and staff not only slows decision-making but also creates large numbers of people with the power to block change.	☐
Prior Experience With Change Score three if the organization has successfully implemented major changes in the recent past. Score one if there is no prior experience with major change or if change efforts failed or left a legacy of anger or resentment. Most companies will score two, acknowledging equivocal success in previous attempts to change.	☐
Morale Change is easier if employees enjoy working in the organization and the level of individual responsibility is high. Signs of unreadiness to change: low team spirit, little voluntary extra effort, and mistrust. Look for two types of mistrust: between management and employees, and between or among departments.	☐

Innovation Best situation: The company is always experimenting; new ideas are implemented with seemingly little effort; employees work across internal boundaries without much trouble. Bad signs: lots of red tape, multiple signoffs required before new ideas are tried; employees must go through channels and are discouraged from working with colleagues from other departments or divisions.	☐
Decision-Making Rate yourself high if decisions are made quickly, taking into account a wide variety of suggestions; it is clear where decisions are made. Give yourself a low grade if decisions come slowly and are made by a mysterious "them"; there is a lot of conflict during the process, and confusion and finger pointing after decisions are announced.	☐
Total Score	☐

Table 5.5. Quiz to test an organization's readiness for change.[11]   (© 1993 Time Inc. All rights reserved.)

Evaluate your organizations total score according to the scale shown in Table 5.6. Do not focus on the total score only. The quiz also helps identify the specific organizational problem areas that may need to be addressed *prior* to the change effort itself.

Conclusion

In talking with change leaders and information system implementers around the world, we have heard over and over, "My situation is unique!" We agree that the people, the resources, and the exact details of each situation are unique; still, there are some organizational behavioral characteristics that are rather common. People throughout the world have similar needs for involvement and interaction. This chapter was designed to help change leaders link together basic organizational principles to basic human organizational interactions. In your "unique" situation, the time to think about your organizational issues is before beginning the informatics implementation. What organizational strategies and tactics will be necessary to lessen the resistance to change and move

Total Score	Interpretation
41–51	Implementing change is most likely to succeed. Focus resources on lagging factors (your ones and twos) to accelerate the process.
28–40	Change is possible but may be difficult, especially if you have low scores in the first seven readiness dimensions. Bring those up to speed before attempting to implement large-scale change.
17–27	Implementing change will be virtually impossible without a precipitating catastrophe. Focus instead on (1) building change readiness in the dimensions above and (2) effecting change through skunkworks or pilot programs separate from the organization at large.

Table 5.6. Quiz to test an organization's readiness for change.[11]   (© 1993 Time Inc. All rights reserved.)

your informatics systems forward for the benefit of your overall organization?

In the following chapter, we will look at the first step in the change process, the establishment of the strategic directions that will provide the basis for the more detailed plans to follow.

Questions

1. Do you think technical people are most comfortable functioning at Katz's "production of goods and services" level of management concerns? Why or why not?
2. Why are quality efforts considered to be proactive rather than reactive?
3. Why is it necessary to understand and assess the global technology issues and environment?
4. Vision—what is it? How do you decide what to include? Where do you begin?
5. What are several ways to minimize the change leaders "point person" role?
6. What organizational strategies and tactics will be necessary to lessen the resistance to technological changes?

References

1. Katz, RL. Skills of an effective administrator. In: *Harvard Business Review: On Management.* New York: Harper & Row, 1975;19–34.
2. Boyett, JH, Conn, HP. *Workplace 2000: The Revolution Reshaping American Business.* New York: Dutton, 1991.
3. Naisbitt, J. *Megatrends: Ten New Directions Transforming Our Lives.* New York: Warner Books, 1982.
4. Alsop, S. Distributed thinking. *Infoworld* September 27, 1993;4.
5. Baum, D. Case study: Health-care firm heals its data management woes. *Infoworld* January 17, 1994;62.
6. Holmes, B. The impact of clinical information systems on the future of nursing. *NSNA/Imprint* February-March, 1990;39–40.
7. Van Kirk, D. Client/server creates challenges, opportunities. *Infoworld* December 13, 1993;50.
8. Tannenbaum, R, Schmidt, WH. How to choose a leadership pattern. *Harvard Business Review* 1958;36(March-April):877–917.
9. Lorenzi, NM. Making the dream come true: Role of the medical school library. *Bulletin of the Medical Library Association* 1983;71:410–414.
10. Kanter, RM. *Men and Women of the Corporation.* New York: Basic Books, 1977.
11. Stewart, TA. Rate your readiness to change. *Fortune* February 7,1994, 106–110.

6
Determining the Strategic Direction

Whether in patient care, research, administration, or education, the applications of all types of technologies are exploding in today's health care arena. In patient care, technology is used to admit patients to a hospital, order their tests, perform their tests (e.g., in radiology and laboratory procedures), disseminate the test results, maintain their medical records, provide feedback to the referring physician, followup on patients in ambulatory sites, etc. Technology today can suggest treatment modalities in medicine and surgery. Technology is increasingly integrating the patient into the health care decision process. Using technology, patients can explore both the available treatment options and the potential outcomes to help them make more informed treatment choices. In essence, the infrastructure of the modern health care world has shifted from bricks and mortar to technology.

The support of research through technology is also growing. Without computers, the mapping of the human genome would never have been undertaken in the first place, let alone have a completion date far ahead of the initial expectation. This type of research effort will produce a second-order–type change in the "practice" of medicine. There will be a time when patients can be "mapped" to determine future disease states and to "genetically treat" those states before they occur.

In the past, the decision, application, and management of technology resources were issues of organizational debate and discussion. In a surprising number of cases, there was little or no integration or coordination of the informatics strategies with the overall organizational strategies. The informatics strategies—if explicitly defined at all—were set in a kind of organizational vacuum, resulting in considerable suboptimization. Today's focus is the management of integrated technologies throughout the organization as a source of sustainable competitive advantage. How, then, does an organization determine its strategic technological direction to further that quest?

Establishing a strategic information direction is the process through which the organization allocates its scarce information technology resources to achieve outcomes that satisfy the organization's constituencies. Therefore, the strategic informatics direction can be defined as the allocation of information technology resources (machines, software, personnel, etc.) to enable the organization to achieve its goals.

Why have a strategy? Many organizations have a vague implicit strategy that the leadership typically claims that everyone knows, understands, and completely accepts. Believing this ranks right with belief in the Tooth Fairy. An explicit, carefully crafted, widely communicated strategic informatics plan is essential if the organization expects to hold people accountable for making intelligent, coordinated resource decisions. Different organizations need different informatics strategies. Like people, no two organizations are exactly alike, so no two informatics strategies should be alike in detail. It is critical that the strategic informatics direction incorporates the realities of the particular organization and its overall organizational strategies.

Strategic Guiding Informatics Principles

When Alice asked the Cheshire cat for directions, the cat asked her destination. Alice answered that the destination didn't much matter, and the cat replied that it then wouldn't make much difference which way she went. Before trying to create detailed plans for an informatics thrust, the organization needs to develop some strategic guiding informatics principles. While we often jokingly refer to these as "suitable for framing," they do have a definite purpose. These principles should convey the broad informatics aims against which subsequent, more specific plans can be interpreted, judged, and modified if necessary. These principles can also be useful to those people caught in situations in which decisions become bogged down in politics, territoriality, etc. The following examples of broad guiding principles might be appropriate for many health care organizations if they match the organization's values and overall directional philosophy.

Example 1

"The implementation of all technology within our institution must be seamless regardless of the physical location of the information, its perceived ownership, or the organizational structure involved." This example illustrates a thrust for an organization-wide systems approach as opposed to allowing information fiefdoms to continue or even grow.

Example 2

"Our strategic technological decisions must integrate our customers' needs and the organization's internal processes and systems to gain a competitive advantage." This example illustrates the issue of focusing efforts on customer needs rather than the traditional focus on producer activities. The competitive advantage reference is designed to stress the point that we are in competition and that if we don't satisfy our customers' needs, someone else will.

Example 3

"Our information technology management process must be totally integrated from the idea stage through final implementation to ensure the delivery of higher value added outcomes for customers." This example focuses on the quality of the development process, encouraging team or "concurrent" development processes as opposed to traditional stage-to-stage linear hand-off processes. This approach also stresses beginning-to-end responsibility for those involved with a project. The inclusion of the value added concept stresses a criterion against which resources can be allocated.

Example 4

"We must maintain a creative attitude in all our informatics efforts—thinking in long term ways, being flexible, confronting obstacles boldly, thinking broadly, and setting bold targets." This example stresses the importance of long-term thinking and long-term solutions as opposed to an endless series of quick fixes. It also places a value on creativity and innovation versus simple extensions of the status quo.

Example 5

"We must move beyond technology acquisition to the concept of technology assimilation." This example again places the emphasis on outcomes rather than activities. Mere acquisition can lead to an accumulation of incompatible resources; the assimilation concept requires taking a total systems point of view with all that view implies such as end-user and customer satisfaction.

Key Questions to Ask

Both the technical literature and the daily newspapers are filled with the latest "gee whiz" technologies and their amazing supposed capabilities. These, however, are simply the *tools* for implementing our information strategies. If we have developed and implemented sound information principles, these will help us greatly in determining which of the available technology paths we should follow and at what rate. Here are some key questions that need to be answered as we develop the information principles and strategies appropriate to our particular organization.

- Who are the current "champions" for the development of explicit strategic principles?
- Who else's early support is critical, and how do we get it?
- What are the time constraints for the development of these strategic principles?
- What are the relevant historical factors?
- What will be the most effective processes to use in developing these principles?
- Who should be involved?
- What are the organizational plans that must be considered in developing strategic directions?
- What is the role of the chief information officer (whether formally designated as such or not) in determining the strategic principles?
- What practical political factors have to be considered?
- Once the principles are determined, how can additional agreement and support be obtained?
- What other events need to happen for the successful establishment of new information principles?

Once answers are sought to these questions, other questions will also arise to provide us with the information we need. This set of questions should serve to start the process.

Relationship to Overall Planning

How do these strategic information principles relate to what we normally think of as the planning process? Many organizations have regular planning cycles such as five-year plans or annual plans in addition to project planning for particular projects. Figure 6.1 shows the structure we recommend for the overall planning process in the health informatics area.

The strategic information principles serve as the foundation for the three planning levels that follow. At each higher level, the plan is more detailed and the time horizon is shorter. If a poor job is done at any level, the prices are typically paid over and over at the higher levels. For example, if we never clearly determine whether our strategic direction will be toward seamless systems integration (see Example 1, above) then proponents of alternative strategies will fight this battle every time a new implementation occurs. Further, the summation of these individual battles does not typically produce a strategy. The normal outcome is continual organizational strife and wasted information resources.

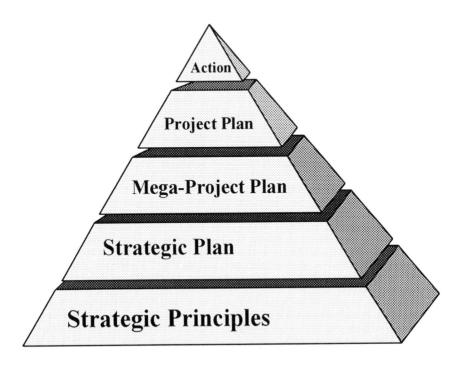

Figure 6.1. The overall planning process for the health informatics area.

Overall Planning Process Example

The lower-level foundations in Figure 6.1 become the source of the more detailed and timely plans at the higher levels. Inverting the pyramid, the impact of the principles cascades downward, creating more detailed plans at each level. At the same time, detailed plans must support—or at least not conflict with in major ways—all the strategic steps. The following is an example of how the four planning levels in Figure 6.1 might mesh.

- *Strategic principles.* Assume that a hospital adopts the seamless integration principle (Example 1, above) as one of its strategic information principles.
- *Strategic plan.* Among a wide range of other aspects, the strategic plan might state that (1) the hospital will adopt a unified database model for the entire organization and that (2) no new technologies—information or medical—will be allowed that do not support two-way communication with this database model. This strategy might well be supportive of strategic principles other than just the seamless integration one.
- *Mega-project plan.* How will the strategic plan be implemented? The mega-project plan could specify a process for developing the institution-wide database model, a general plan for implementing the model across the institution, and a process for ensuring that new technologies fit the model.
- *Project plan.* The project plans are the situation-specific detailed plans to actually implement the above broader plans. In this case, an example might be to convert the existing systems in the radiology department to conform to our new database model. Another example might be a system selection project to test a proposed piece of automated lab equipment for information compatibility with the new model. The implementation of the mega-project plan could include hundreds of these project plans, and a particular project plan could support several if not all of the strategic principles.

Does all this planning activity take time? It certainly does—lots of it. However, as the old planning cliché states, "We don't plan to fail; we only fail to plan!" For action-oriented people, it is almost impossible to expend quality time on the planning processes to the point where the marginal value is negative. The bias toward action will almost always stop the planning process while additional time spent would still result in more time saved in subsequent stages than spent in the additional planning.

Some Critical Health Informatics Planning Issues

There are four key issues that anyone doing planning in the health informatics areas must constantly keep in mind and also communicate effectively to others in the organization. Today, people throughout the organization read constantly about new technologies, and many consider themselves well informed in the informatics area—whether they are or not. Effective communications to these amateur informaticians is essential if the plans are to be accepted.

Parallelism

From the strategic information principles to the project plans, all health informatics planning must be in parallel with the strategies and plans of the parent organization. While this point may seem self-evident, huge amounts of informatics resources have been wasted by organizational units pursuing their own agendas, whether from ignorance or indifference. Figure 6.2 uses a vector approach to illustrate the point that nonparallel efforts lead to economic waste from the perspective of the overall organization.

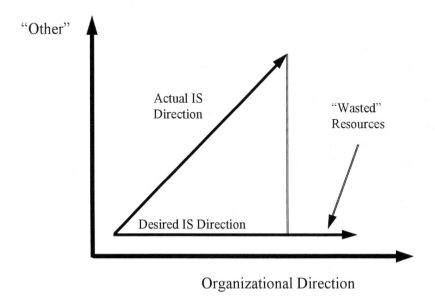

Figure 6.2. The impact of nonparallelism in the information system (IS) planning process.

In Figure 6.2, the horizontal vector labeled Desired IS Direction represents an amount of effort or resources expended in the direction considered appropriate by the overall organization. The upward sloping vector labeled Actual IS Direction shows that all of those IS efforts are unfortunately not going in the "right" direction. Part of the effort is in pursuit of "Other," which might be things that are more interesting, more comfortable, more visible, higher résumé value, etc. Regardless, the impact is shown by the vertical line, which illustrates the amount of progress in the "Organizational Direction." The vector segment labeled "Wasted" Resources illustrates the amount of lost potential progress. What if the Actual IS Direction line were closer to parallel with the Desired IS Direction? The amount of "Wasted" Resources would decrease. If the Actual were even further from the Desired, the "Wasted" Resources would increase rapidly.

The challenge to the management of both the overall organization and the information area is obvious—to maintain constant vigilance that the informatics resources are being spent in the right ways.

Pace of Change

The pace of change in both the medical and information technology areas is very fast. Also astounding in the information area is the pace at which previously separate technologies—the computer, telephones, cable TV, etc.—are being integrated. This fast pace of change and its accompanying high uncertainty make traditional types of leisurely planning relatively useless. More and more the premium is on adaptive plans and planning processes. The most adaptive plan is the plan that allows irrevocable decisions to be made the latest—while maintaining the same ultimate deadline. Typically, there is going to be a price paid for this adaptivity. This price can be thought of as a type of insurance cost in the sense that the price is being paid for risk reduction.

Vendor Misinformation

A practical rule is that the newer the technology, the more inflated and/or misleading the vendor claims will be. In the information area, "vaporware" has become an accepted term for the vendors' promises about product capabilities and delivery dates. This is especially important in strategic planning as various vendors will loudly assert distinctly different visions of the future. As James Abrahamson of Oracle recently said, "Every company out there can define the information highway for you. It's the strategic vision for whatever the company happens to sell."[1] In this industry "buyer beware" is important not only for the actual product but also for the information disseminated well in advance by the vendors.

Installed Base

All planning must always consider the eternal albatross of the informatics area, the organization's installed base of information systems. Except in true cutting-edge areas, one rarely gets the opportunity to start from scratch. We inherit existing practices, databases, software, hardware, etc. Thus, any future directional shift must not only position the organization for the future, but must also accommodate the past. Unfortunately, this often means the sins of the past!

Organizational Planning Styles

Different organizations will inevitably use different styles in developing strategic information plans. No one style can be labeled as best; the style must fit the organization. The planning styles can be grouped into four broad categories:

1. *Top-Down (CEO Driven).* The CEO gathers information, makes the decision, and essentially tells the rest of the organization to get on board or get out.
2. *Middle-In (Whiz Kids).* The middle managers and/or the technical professionals perceive the informatics future with its threats and opportunities and persuade the organization to adopt their plan. This model is not uncommon when you have a combination of a mature organization with older upper management, a rapidly changing technical environment, and good levels of self-esteem within the organization.
3. *Bottom-Up (Entrepreneurial).* In a relatively decentralized system, individuals with initiative create their own systems and the ones that work best—or at least receive the most notice—are adopted for the overall system.
4. *Organizational Emergent (Organizational Learning—Non-Planning Plan).* The organization communicates its goals clearly and then empowers individuals and units to meet the goals, developing the necessary systems on a consensual basis.

Within a larger organization, different units may well use different styles internally. When joint action between units is necessary, the former two will generally prevail over the latter two.

Who Should Be Involved?

Who should be involved in formulating strategic informatics principles and plans? Perhaps the better question is, Who should *not* be involved? The ideal is to maximize to the extent possible the representation of all levels throughout the process. While planning can never be 100 percent participatory, the rule of thumb is, the greater the level of detail, the wider the involvement or participation should be. Only a few people will be involved at the conceptual levels; however, everyone affected should be involved or at least represented at the detail level. Understanding the scale and scope of the impact can be done through stakeholder analysis. Stakeholders are the individuals, groups, and other organizations that will be affected by or can affect the strategic informatics direction and plan. Insights into the barriers and benefits generated by stakeholders are important.

Effective Planning Methods

There are many different types of planning methodologies. All the methodologies provide some type of structured process for the planner to follow. Bradley J. Dixon of the University of Western Ontario contends that there are two very different schools of thought on strategic planning.[2] The structure school of thought, made famous by Prof. Michael Porter, focuses on what factors to consider (for example, how to build barriers to entry to suppress competition). Porter developed a five-forces model, including value chain, competitive value of nations, and others.

The process school, led by Henry Mintzberg, concentrates on the strategy formulation process—it is not what you do, but how you do it. They agree that the structures are important, but they also add a component for how plans are implemented. Unfortunately, most strategic planning frameworks emphasize structure to the exclusion of the process, but the process school is undergoing renewed interest.

The process school of thought concentrates on the issue of understanding how the organization is moving toward whatever goal it is pursuing. Using the vector concept of Figure 6.2, understanding why various unit strategies align with the strategies of the organization and each other is considered more important than the actual direction they are heading. This demonstrates why an average strategy executed in a highly coordinated manner will beat an excellent strategy executed by units pursuing their own agendas. This conclusion is based on the finding that a strategy can be readily copied, whereas the implementation cannot be so easily replicated.

In the Mintzberg and Quinn model, rather than focusing on what the people are currently doing, we set and announce some *intended strategies*.[3] Then we encourage people over time to move in the right direction. However, as changes occur and feedback is received, we modify the strategies as necessary. Through this continuous strategy development process, we may move toward strategies significantly different from the original intended ones. These eventual strategies are called the *realized strategies*.

The Role of the CIO

Chief information officers (CIOs) normally have four areas of responsibility within the organization.

1. *Technical management.* This involves overseeing the actual operations of the information systems function.
2. *Education and communications.* This includes educating and communicating at all levels, above and below, and in all functional areas of the organization. Two important aspects are gradually establishing a common informatics language in the organization and communicating a set of realistic expectations.
3. *Building trust.* Trust is an interesting word in that it can have two meanings that are often not differentiated in casual conversation. One is that I trust your *competence,* your ability to get results. The other is that I trust you as a *person,* referring to your honesty, your ethics, your integrity. When a CIO loses either kind of trust, the meaning of CIO starts to change from "chief information officer" to "career is over!"
4. *Advancing the organizational goals.* This is translating the CEO's and the board's strategic plans for the organization into relevant information technology implementations, and translating somewhat abstract business strategies goals into quite concrete technical activities.

The acid test of a successful CIO is the quality of the CEO/CIO relationship. Brad Dixon suggests that the critical questions for CIOs are, "What specific thing has my CEO done for me (my area) lately? How has my CEO supported or failed to support me (my area) lately?" These are often very telling questions. Both parties may feel they have a fine relationship. After all, they play golf together every weekend. They may even consider themselves as personal friends. However, the acid test is *support*. In a business sense, is the relationship with the CEO functional or dysfunctional? The quality of this relationship may be the single best predictor of the CIO's longevity.

Politics and Planning

The very word *politics* has a negative meaning to many people. In a book such as this, we could try to skirt the issue by using terms such as *organizational processes* or *influence management*. However, these more pleasant euphemisms do not change the basic problem. To achieve successful health informatics implementations, we have to possess reasonable political skills in the organizational sense. Chapter 9 is devoted entirely to the political processes in health informatics. However, we are including a few points here that are relevant to the strategic planning process.

One key in setting strategic information directions is to avoid linking the strategy too closely to a particular individual or political flag. Politics change and CEOs change. Make sure that the policy is appropriate for the time, not just for the person. Most importantly be aware of the political environment. Plans cannot and should not be changed at whim.

Five key areas for building political support for the strategic informatics directions are:

- *Use resources wisely.* Lack of adequate resources can starve any plan. However, the plan must be perceived by key people as using the organization's scarce resources judiciously. We must be able to show that our area is focused on adding value for the organization.
- *Sell the plan.* Of course our plan is brilliant, and anyone should be able to see that. This is looking at the plan through our eyes. They want to know (1) what is in it for them and (2) what is in it for the organization, *in that order*. If there is nothing in it for them, don't expect their support unless you have something else to trade or can call in past favors. We

can argue forever that it should not be that way, but these are the realities of organizational life.

♦ *Manage their expectations.* Promise what you can deliver and deliver what you promise. Don't oversell. Unmet expectations pave the road to the hell of lost credibility.

♦ *Mesh strategic and operational plans.* Informatics must support the operational and strategic plans of other departments and the entire organization. This means that we must first identify and then express their plans in a general sense. We can't integrate what we don't know.

♦ *Make informatics enable strategic organizational change.* Informatics investments rarely provide outstanding returns unless they enable strategic organizational change. Paving the ox cart paths has limited returns. The current interest in reengineering or process redesign is acknowledging the limits to incrementalism that has been a hallmark of many informatics plans. Understand how the strategic informatics direction will enable strategic change and work toward realizing the change.

Conclusion

Strategic planning is only the beginning. If we do a good job, our health informatics efforts will integrate with our organization's overall thrusts. In addition, a sound planning process will have begun the task of building support for and ownership in our plans. Finally, nothing about the plans or the planning process is cast in stone. Both the plans and the process must be dynamic, ready to change to meet changing needs and conditions. However, we implement at tactical levels, not strategic ones. In the next chapter, we examine the next level of detail in the preimplementation process.

Questions

1. Why do organizations need a technology strategy, since technology changes so rapidly?
2. Why are "champions" essential for implementing a technology strategy?
3. Who should be involved in formulating strategic informatics principles and plans? What should be the role of the chief information officer in determining the strategic direction? The chief executive officer?

4. To what extent does an organization's history or past place limits upon its current vision for the future and strategic directions? Explain.

References

1.   Reinhardt, A. Building the data highway. *Byte* 1994;3:46–74.
2.   *Draft Proceedings of the International Medical Informatics Association Working Conference on the Organizational Impact of Informatics.* Cincinnati: Riley Associates, 1993.
3.   Mintzberg, H. Crafting strategy. *Harvard Business Review* 1987; July-August:66–75.

7
Some Critical Issues in Project Planning and Management

The development of strategic directions discussed in Chapter 6 is critical for long-term success. However, the actual implementation process requires far more detailed communication and planning. The managerial framework used for health informatics implementations is typically the one known as *project management*. This is not a book on the details and techniques of project management; there are already many good ones on the market. For those needing a managerial primer on the subject, we recommend *Project Management* by Meredith and Mantel.[1]

Despite all the books and seminars on the topic, sound project management is still more the exception than the rule. The following piece of anonymous photocopier graffiti, "The Six Phases of a Project," can be found posted somewhere on the wall in virtually every project environment.

1. Wild enthusiasm.
2. Intense disillusionment.
3. Mindless panic.
4. A desperate search for the guilty.
5. Cruel and unusual punishment of the innocent.
6. Praise and honors heaped upon the nonparticipants.

The sardonic nature of the humor—and even bitterness—contained in the above is obvious. Many people have been involved in informatics projects that can best be described as less than well managed—to put it kindly. Anyone charged with managing a major implementation often has to overcome an initial attitude of cynicism among those involved.

There are several particular aspects of planning and managing a health care informatics project that do intersect heavily with the people and organizational issues that are the focus of this book.

If you are not familiar with technical projects and their peculiarities, we strongly urge you to read Tracy Kidder's book, *The*

Soul of a New Machine,[2] for which Kidder won a Pulitzer Prize in 1982. The details of the particular project described by Kidder are not that important; the value of the book is in the descriptions of the pressures, the motivations, and the ups and downs of a major technical project. It is a unique book and well worth reading.

In this chapter, some of the focus is on the internal operations or aspects of the project; however, at virtually every step, these internal aspects either interact with the project environment or have an impact on the relations with that environment sooner or later.

Traditional Information Systems Development

We begin by looking at how traditional information systems projects have been conducted and then look at concepts and approaches that can overcome many of the traditional shortcomings.

Worst-Case Scenario

A relatively haughty techie descends from Olympus and interviews the manager of an area to find out how the work of that area is done. This approach fails to recognize that any manager of more than six people who has had the position for more than one year typically *does not know how the system really works.* The manager knows how it *should* work and perhaps even does work for typical cases. The reality in our organizations is that good people often make poor systems work by giving special handling to exceptions and special cases. Using the top-down approach, the techie learns virtually nothing about the many potential exceptions.

The techie returns to Olympus and the pantheon of techno-gods work their wonders. A major system is produced and implemented, usually using programming tools that have the flexibility of cast iron. Then the fun begins as the system fails to handle anything but the most mundane transactions. At this point, the finger-pointing begins in earnest. In many cases, the techies defend their system vigorously and "suggest" that the people be forced to adapt to it. Another alternative is that a manual system is quietly run in parallel with the electronic system so the people can actually get their work done. They find it easier to duplicate than fight.

Worst Case with Chrome Plating

In this case, the techie talks to the front-line people as well as to the manager. Now the techie does learn about *some* of the exceptions and current special procedures. Rarely, however, does the user remember anywhere near all of them, and the techie is rarely a skilled-enough interviewer to draw them all out. From here the process proceeds the same as above. The results do tend to be somewhat more acceptable since at least some of the exceptions—one hopes the major ones—have been handled. Also, the end user does feel some ownership as there has been at least some participation. However, the process still tends to produce cast-iron solutions with little flexibility.

Worst Case with Gold Plating

Now the IS people decide to modernize their approach. They buy a sophisticated, expensive CASE (computer aided software engineering) system to add discipline, structure, and organization to their development process, and the appropriate IS people are extensively trained at great expense. Yet, in many cases, the CASE system ends up on the shelf.[3] The basic problem is that these CASE tools do not effectively address the part of the development process that causes the most problem—the determination of what the end user really needs. Tools such as CASE merely refine the traditional inadequate process.

A More Modern Approach

The modern approach focuses much more strongly on what the user needs from the system and the best way for the user to interface with the system. In this approach, software is used that provides rapid prototyping capabilities, allowing the techie to quickly create a prototype of the system as he or she currently understands it at any stage. It is immediately shown to the prospective users who try it. Often, some of the user's complaints or suggestions can be implemented on the spot; others may require the techie to create another version. Using this team developmental approach usually lengthens some of the early development steps; however, overall development time is typically reduced significantly, for obvious reasons. Perhaps just as important, the tools used in this approach tend to provide systems that are far more flexible than those produced by traditional approaches.

Those unfamiliar with traditional IS approaches may not realize how culturally significant the transition is for an IS area to move to this last model. The traditional approaches are very consistent with the information politics model of technocratic utopianism discussed in Chapter 4; therefore, moving from it involves significant cultural change.

Product Development Analogy

Business Week magazine conducted an extensive study of new product developments to determine some of the reasons for failure.[4] Most of their examples focused on physical product failures such as RCA's videodisk or IBM's PC jr. As a study outcome, *Business Week* developed the six guidelines presented below.[5] We found it interesting to see how closely this physical product example related to some of the needs of "new product development" in the health care informatics area.

"Ask Your Customers"

Customers have needs they want met. Or if it is a very innovative product, they want to know, "What will it do for me?" Techies love *features,* customers want *benefits!* A classic example of this is the failure of most of the flashy interactive kiosk projects that have been attempted.[6] They only tend to work when the user wants very detailed information or precise services. Otherwise, humans prefer to ask other humans quick questions and get quick answers.

"Set Realistic Goals"

Failure can be guaranteed if the goals are set too high. Don't saddle a potentially fine product with overly glamorous predictions.

"Break Down Walls"

Use integrated teams to achieve best results. Using traditional "hand-off" models in which each area works on something and then hands it to another area, leads to low ownership throughout the process.

"Create Gateways"

Create gateways or checkpoints at which each project is reviewed for current status and continued desirability. One of the classic economic principles is that sunk costs are irrelevant. Once we have spent resources, they are lost. The question to be addressed is whether we should spend the required future dollars on this project. Don't let inertia dictate continued funding of a dog.

"Watch Those Tests"

Testing can be deceptive for a variety of reasons, especially if the amount of data is limited. If in doubt at key stages, test some more, especially if the costs of a misstep are high.

"Do Your Postmortems"

Managers tend to run away from their failures. Don't. Formally review what went wrong and apply those lessons to the next launch. Reward managers who learn from mistakes.

Project Management for System Implementation

Modern information technology is far more than a collection of wires, resistors, "chips," plastic, and sheet metal. It is the productive combination of hardware, software, and human and environmental factors. Implementing information technology is as much as social process as a technical one. People who are oriented to thinking of technology solely in hardware—or even software—terms have a hard time appreciating the emotional reactions that technological change issues often provoke.

One central theme is that the road to successful technology implementation must have—like any good road—a solid foundation or under-structure before the paving begins. In this case, that foundation is a total systems approach involving planning, planning, and more planning. To many action or task-oriented people, the thought of all this planning time is appalling. They may give lip service to planning, but their actions reflect their true belief—planning is a waste of precious time that could be used for implementation. Unfortunately, there are countless horror stories of poor planning leading to bungled implementations of technology.

A total systems approach is also critical, which means two things: (1) the use of a reasonably extensive project management model to provide discipline and structure to the complete technology transfer process, and (2) an exhaustive search for *all* of the relevant variables to consider and/or include in the total project management process.

The Project Management Process

Projects and the project management process can be viewed in many ways depending upon the perspective of the viewer. The following set of issues is one we have found useful in analyzing the success and failure of health informatics projects of any size. Some of the comments below will be elaborated upon subsequently.

Definition of Responsibilities

An army must have one commanding general; a project must have one person in charge. While this person may report to a "board of directors" in a policy sense, the operational authority and responsibility must be with this one person. In the same way, the responsibility for each distinct project step must be assigned to one person. This does not imply in any way that the project leadership needs to be autocratic or authoritarian. It means that the lines of communication and responsibility need to be clearly defined.

A major question in a hospital environment always seems to be, Who is (should be) in charge? If the project is technically driven, a "technical type" is usually in charge; if it is to be applications driven, a functional person such as a pharmacist is in charge. Until these responsibility issues are resolved, it is pointless to proceed, regardless of the political and managerial conflicts these assignments may raise.

Objective Setting

The first step in managing the project must be the setting of realistic objectives. Further, all of the significant parties involved must have some definite emotional commitment or ownership in these objectives. The question is, Who are the people or groups who will be affected by this new system? Without some degree of ownership from them, subsequent negotiations and problem solving will be both prolonged and frustrating to everyone involved. Obtaining extensive early ownership is usually a very participative, time-consuming process that has a very high payoff during the implementation stage. The final objectives should include specific, realistic definitions of project success. Again, until this stage is completed, no further work should proceed.

Action Planning

The action steps required for project success should first be defined in terms of ten to twenty major steps with start and end dates established for each step. Then the planning process should move to the next lower level of detail, again following the general pattern of defining ten to twenty steps. As successively lower levels of detail are reached, input should be actively sought from the people responsible for eventually implementing that part of the plan. This is critical to obtain both their valuable input and their psychological commitment. Always remember that it is virtually impossible for action-oriented people to "overplan," i.e., to reach the point of negative marginal returns from the planning process.

Tight Control/Feedback Procedures

An organized system must be designed and put into place to obtain timely feedback on the status of each portion of the project. It is critical to obtain the earliest possible warning of any deviations from schedule or budget—positive or negative. In this managerial context, the word *control* refers to controlling the *system*, not controlling people in some negative sense.

Ongoing Problem Solving

Unforeseen problems arise in virtually every project, although quality planning does help reduce them. As problems do arise, they must be dealt with by a problem-solving approach—not a finger-pointing one. The project manager's responsibility is to keep a positive general atmosphere. Finger pointing and "blaming" simply lead to negativism, defensiveness, and the temptation to seek revenge—all fatal to project success.

Project Completion

As the project approaches completion, an evaluation process should begin to measure the success of the project against the original success criteria. This process will both provide feedback to the supporters or funders and provide feedback to the project team. The first should be mandatory, and the second is simply good management. In most organizations, valuable experience gained from one project is not made easily available to those with similar or related subsequent projects. Thus, the wheel is eternally reinvented.

Some Critical Project Concepts

We have had years of experience with projects of all sizes and types and even have some organizational "scars" from these experiences. On a positive note, we have also learned some ways of preventing or reducing the many types of problems that can arise in implementing complex health informatics projects. The following are key concepts that we think will work for you.

- Put in ample time and energy up front.
- Set realistic system performance objectives.
- Set realistic systems development expectations.
- Plan, plan, and plan some more.
- Use team approaches.
- Build flexible systems.
- Manage the key project values well.
- Constantly improve your management processes.

Let us look at these key concepts and some tools and guidelines for implementing them.

Put in Ample Time and Energy Up Front

"You can pay me now or you can pay me later!" In a classic TV commercial for automobile oil filters, a grease-covered mechanic used these words to tout the advantage of replacing oil filters regularly. He threatened that if you didn't choose to spend a few dollars now on preventing problems, you would have to spend a lot more money later in repairing those problems. If anything, the value of this philosophy is even higher in the case of project management than it is with auto engines. If there is any one message that summarizes this chapter, it is this: moments, hours, or days spent productively at the front of a project in planning, team building, communicating, etc., can literally save days, weeks, or months later in a large project.

Resolve Basic Conflicts Early

In the rush to get started "doing" on a major project, critical conflict issues are often left unresolved. These conflicts might be between implementation team members, between the team and other stakeholders, or between various stakeholders besides the team. It could be conflicts over preferred technical approaches or over the appropriate balance between ease-of-access and security/confidentiality. If these conflicts are not resolved early in the process, they will be fought out in constant guerrilla actions throughout the project. More important, these guerrilla actions typically do not resolve the conflict; they merely perpetuate it. In a war, trading minor defeats and victories typically does not produce a winner or a loser; it just drains the energy and resources of *all* the parties involved. Incidentally, this constant fighting can also quickly kill the enthusiasm of third parties forced either to observe the process or to take sides.

The Japanese with their more group-oriented culture seem to handle this area of early conflict resolution much better than most Western cultures do. The Japanese approach is typically more consensus seeking. The underlying assumption is that when team members can't agree on a particular approach, there is probably either poor communication or a valid problem with that approach. Therefore, let's talk about it some more. On the other hand, Americans tend to use a very different approach. Schooled in individualism and democracy, we "settle" things by majority rule whether or not a formal vote is ever taken. Those who perceive themselves to be in the minority on an issue usually quit arguing and "go along" with the majority. The problem, however, is the minority's lack of ownership in the process. The minority's attitude is often, "All right, let's see you make *your* idea work!" or gleeful finger pointing if the majority's idea fails.

As a general rule, the consensus building approaches take quite a bit more time up front, but the subsequent implementation process is rapid. Many problems have been foreseen and solved in advance or prevented from occurring. Also, ownership and motivation tend to be high. The "voting" approach tends to lead to quicker starts, but leaves more issues and problems to be resolved downstream in the implementation process. Some argue that the latter approach is also more conducive to creativity. To the extent that is true, the price in stress and wasted resources is high.

Set Realistic System Performance Objectives

In an informatics implementation, the expectations fall into two broad areas:

- the performance of the system that is developed in terms of its ability to meet organizational needs and satisfy the end users
- the quality of the implementation process in terms of meeting time, budget, and technical specifications.

How Results are Judged

Whether we are talking about system performance or the development process, our overall results are the comparison of performance to expectations or objectives. Dismal performance on either dimension can be the source of poor results. In many real-world situations, however, the problem of so-called poor results may stem more from the expectations side than the performance side. Case A in Figure 7.1 depicts the situation in which the expectations (of either type) were set at a realistic level and the subsequent actual performance matched the expectation. This is the type of result that we should be considering as normal in our organizations.

Case B is a surprisingly common type of situation in many poorly managed technical areas. Here, expectations are set at a quite unrealistic level, and the system then struggles to achieve the impossible. The performance may well be quite decent, i.e., meeting a realistic expectation; however, the general feeling is often one of, "Well, I guess you didn't do too badly but . . ." Something is wrong here when good performance receives marginal feedback.

Case C represents the outcome that a potential Case B situation can easily slide toward. Sound psychology tells us that targets should be *realistic* and *challenging,* but *attainable.* When targets are imposed that the implementers perceive as unattainable, they tend to set their own internal, unstated targets which may be considerably lower than the "official" ones. This can lead to performance that is relatively poor, especially in comparison to the original exaggerated expectations. The overall results are a significant blow to the credibility of the implementers.

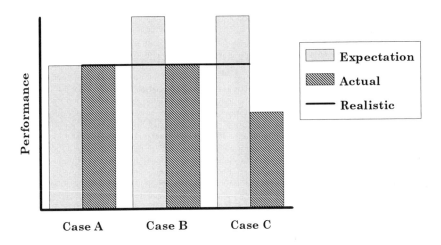

Figure 7.1. Alternative performance cases—expected versus actual.

We first discuss the issue of system performance expectations and then look at implement process expectations. American folk history tells us that a visitor to President Theodore Roosevelt saw the president's small dog limp into the room, bloody and battered. The visitor commented that it was a shame that the dog was not a better fighter. Roosevelt replied that the dog was an excellent fighter but, unfortunately, was a very poor judge of other dogs. We doubt that most of our organizations would be so tolerant in forming their opinions of our performance and abilities. In a quality organization, management is going to expect the leaders of health informatics efforts to:

1. set target levels for system performance that are realistic, challenging, and attainable, and then
2. meet or exceed these target levels unless there are obvious extenuating circumstances.

Why is this worth discussing? It seems so obvious or "just common sense." Without specific measures, the judgment of success or failure becomes a purely subjective exercise based upon personal opinions and biases.

One of the management concepts we use in seminars is "the sheep and the wolves." The sheep in organizations are the risk and conflict avoiders whose basic credo is, "Never face up to a risk or conflict today that can be put off until tomorrow."[7] When faced with the prospect of setting explicit expectations—with their implied accountability—sheep typically react in one of three ways:

- trying even under pressure to include loopholes or areas of vagueness in the expectations,
- trying to get agreement to expectations so low that virtually anyone would be guaranteed to meet them,
- agreeing to completely unrealistic expectations imposed from above even though they know these expectations can never be met.

There are obvious negative implications to each of these strategies; however, each traces back to the basic sheep attitude. Let us examine some of the key aspects of setting and communicating quality expectations.

The Importance of Baseline Data

The purpose of new systems is to increase the capabilities for improved performance within the organization. It is critical to have good data on the actual performance capabilities—both as to type and amount—of the current system. These baseline data can provide information that is helpful in two ways:

- it can provide a reality check for us against what we hope the new system can do,
- it can protect us against future unrealistic tales of how good the old system really was.

Anecdotes only go so far. We need solid data upon which to build estimates of improvement and upon which to build support for our new systems on a cost/benefit basis.

The Initial Productivity Curve

Assume that a new system has just been implemented on a ward or in a clinic. Everyone has great expectations for immediate improvements in productivity. However, as the actual implementation begins, the staff's productivity abruptly goes down! Not only does productivity decline, but conflicts possibly arise and working relationships may start to deteriorate. People may begin purposely avoiding or "bad-mouthing" the system. They may well want to return to the "good old days" when things were easier to do, productivity was higher, and they all got along with each other.

Horak[8] suggests that Figure 7.2 depicts the fairly typical relationship between productivity and time as new health informatics systems are implemented. This graph clearly shows the need for carefully managing expectations prior to any significant systems implementation. Horak developed this graph based upon experiences in implementing integrated information systems at five hospitals. In each case, the same general curve pattern held true. Point A represents the level of productivity at the time of initial implementation. Point B is the nadir in productivity, and point C represents the point at which original productivity is regained and improvement finally begins. The duration of times between these points and the magnitudes of the changes varied considerably among the five sites. However, the basic concept depicted by the curve was present in all five cases.

There can be various reasons for the temporary productivity losses such as time spent on the following types of activities:

- training and self-learning on the new system,
- time spent adjusting to new procedures and working relationships,
- time spent dealing with unrelated preexisting problems surfaced by the change process,
- time spent overcoming resistance to the change, perhaps by respected clinicians or other informal leaders who are vocal against the system,

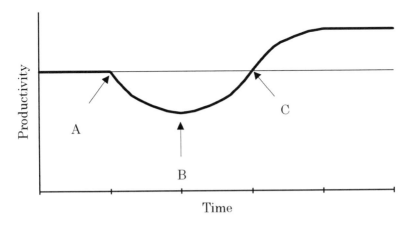

Figure 7.2. System productivity at various times in implementation process.[8]

♦   time spent calming the anxieties and fears of loss of security, autonomy, control, or respect and self-esteem if the system is not quickly mastered.

Taken together, these forces fuel the trauma and decline. Eventually, as the training takes effect and the organizational and psychosocial issues are dealt with, productivity begins to improve and, one hopes, passes presystem levels.

Managing Expectations

In a personal conversation years ago, Jim Scott, an information systems executive for Procter and Gamble, made the following comment, "I constantly preach to my internal consultants that your job is to meet your client's every expectation—after you have first *managed those expectations to realistic levels.*" This is a critical point. If we do not manage our clients' expectations, we are taking a great risk that we will be held to unrealistic expectations they have assembled from who knows where. This also clearly implies that a major role is *client education,* especially when publications from the daily newspaper to *Fortune* to *Modern Maturity* all carry "gee whiz" articles on information technology. More important, these articles typically imply that the technologies described are readily available or "just around the corner." Any systems we produce using reasonably proven technologies are bound to suffer in comparison unless we perform that education well.

Set Realistic Systems Development Expectations

As mentioned in Chapter 1, many information systems departments have developed the reputation that everything they do takes twice as long, costs twice as much, and is half as good as they promised. Once established, this tarnished halo is very difficult to repolish. Yet credibility is a key issue in building and maintaining a successful health informatics program. Establishing realistic systems development expectations and then meeting them is a critical success skill.

Role of Personality

Basic personality plays a large role in the average accuracy of completion time estimates, and Figure 7.3 helps illustrate this point. Assume that the distribution of times to carry out certain tasks is roughly as shown, a bell-shaped curve in this example. The average time that any one task can be expected to take lies under the center of the curve. However, when the following three personalities make their estimates, they effectively view the situation differently at the emotional level.

- The *optimist* or *entrepreneur* focuses on the left side of the curve remembering all the times that tasks like this went smooth as silk. "Why I bet we can knock that out in . . ." The optimist's estimates tend to be repeatedly low, resulting in consistent overcommitment and problems in meetings those commitments. The optimists' teams often tend to be productive; however, the stress price is often high for everyone involved and quality sometimes suffers.
- The *realist* focuses on the midrange of the curve, which appropriately is the realistic part on average. The realist remembers both the easy ones and the hard ones and has a sense of balance. Over time, the realist's estimates average close to reality.
- The *pessimist* or *bureaucrat* is the opposite of the optimist, focusing on the right side of the curve. "Why I can remember some of those that took as long as . . ." The danger with the pessimistic approach is that projects can end up with cost estimates so high that the projects cannot gain approval. Another danger is the Parkinson effect, work expanding to fill available time.

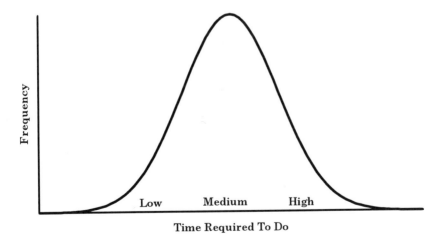

Figure 7.3. Distribution of task completion times.

It is critical that we know where we tend to fall on this spectrum and that we rapidly assess where our associates tend to fall. We all know where vendors in the information industry invariably fall.

Making Realistic Estimates

Few organizations make any attempt to maintain databases of past systems development activities to assist in making realistic time and resource estimates. It is more common to see organizations perpetuate past misestimates than it is to see them learn from past realities. This is tragic but true. Past results may be imperfect predictors of future results, but they at least can provide reality checks for our future activities. Using Figure 7.3 again, our total time and resource estimates should be a summation of midrange estimates or expected values in the words of the statistician. We should not be summing either best-case or worst-case estimates.

When predicting times and resources is difficult, i.e., the uncertainty is high, it is usually quite valuable to use a group approach. Social science research has repeatedly shown that small groups arrive at better solutions of ill-defined amorphous problems than individuals do. Often some sort of Delphi or modified Delphi approach works well. As an example, we have used the following set of steps in the past:

1. have a rough definition of the problem prepared,
2. select a small group of people, e.g., four to seven, that have an interest in the issue,
3. ask the people to independently write down their "answers" or estimates without any prior discussion,
4. make all the answers known to the group without identifying the sources,
5. ask the people to again write down their estimates—the same or different—without any discussion,
6. identify the outlying estimates and ask the authors to discuss, not defend, their reasoning,
7. ask the people to again write down their estimates—the same or different,
8. identify the outlying estimates and ask the authors to discuss, not defend, their reasoning,
9. repeat the two prior steps a few times, if necessary.

This process in practice is not nearly so cumbersome and time-consuming as it appears in writing. It often moves quite rapidly toward a consensus solution. Moreover, there are two major advantages in using this process: the outlier processing provides an opportunity for potential problems or ideas to be raised and integrated into the estimates, and those involved in the process tend to acquire definite ownership in the estimates that are developed by the process.

The Dangers of Overselling

In the words of Robert Service, "For a promise made is a debt unpaid." Therefore, one of the most dangerous strategies is the overselling of a proposed system by either overstating its capabilities or understating its development time and costs. The strategy is often tempting because we know our cause is noble. The organization really "needs" this system, and we may feel that overselling it is the only way to get it approved. This is extremely short-term thinking; we are bound to fail in the sense of meeting expectations and will lose just that much more credibility.

The tragedy is when overselling and guaranteed failure becomes an ingrained part of the organizational culture such as in the way the United States Navy used to get the funding for new ships approved by Congress. The Navy would deliberately understate the costs by a huge amount so that Congress could comfortably give its approval in a political sense. The shipbuilding companies knew to submit low initial bids to support the Navy's underestimates with the under-the-table assurance that they would be allowed to get healthy later on overpriced change orders.

Unfortunately, similar systems have evolved in many companies regarding the costs and other projections surrounding information systems. One side inflates the estimates; the other side discounts them. Where is reality? The problem is a complete loss of meaningful, accurate data for both planning and subsequent performance evaluation. Overselling is ultimately a fool's strategy.

Allowing for Organizational Delays

One of the most common errors in making estimates and plans is failing to allow for delays imposed by organizational issues or friction. The overall organization does not usually see our project as its only important concern. When key approvals, authorizations, reviews, etc., are required, we often find that the key people are caught up in unrelated crises and don't have the time for us right then. Still, we are going to be held accountable for these delays;

therefore it is critical that we don't make unrealistic estimates of how responsive the system will be to our needs.

When Top-Down Limits are Imposed

Management comes to you with an eighteen-month job and says, "We have to have this in twelve months." You say, "I'm sorry, we can't do it in twelve months without a lot more staff." You are then told, "You will have this done in twelve months with your current resources—or we will get somebody who can." What do you do? While many of these situations are not quite so dramatic, the general issue is common; someone with power over us pressures us to do the impossible. We would suggest a few issues to think about and a few strategies to try.

A very compelling question is, "Why is this happening?" One not too pleasant explanation is that the power person does not think much of you in a professional sense. Your estimate of eighteen months merits no respect in this person's eyes. Another alternative is that this person has a neo-fascist management style and believes that impossible goals motivate people. A third possibility is that this person is also under pressure from above and is merely passing that pressure down or on. These are serious issues involving credibility and respect and merit some serious investigation and thought.

What can we do? The most obvious alternative, giving in and promising the impossible, is also a highly undesirable one for numerous reasons. Any more proactive strategies require one thing—good data and plans even if those plans may contain numerous assumptions. Good plans will not necessarily solve the problem, but a lack of plans will typically doom you. If there are data to discuss, this gives an opportunity to move away from the "Yes, you can!" "No, we can't" type of debate, which can only be resolved on a power basis, i.e., you lose.

An assertive strategy we have found useful over the years consists of the following steps.

1. Review your data closely.
2. Make realistic concessions when appropriate.
3. Maintain your poise. Keep the conversation pleasant and professional.
4. Assuming the unrealistic demands continue, smile pleasantly and say, "I'm sorry, but it's not going to happen. Would you like me to lie to you and tell you that it will. I can do that but it still is not going to happen."
5. Be quiet and force a response.

6. If necessary, maintain your poise and keep repeating the above two steps, paraphrasing if necessary to avoid sounding like a parrot.

This process will force some sort of closure other than the original demands. There is no guarantee that you will be completely happy with the outcome; however, it was a quite negative situation to begin with.

Dealing with Those Add-On Requests

Another type of problem, the add-on request, commonly arises in one of two ways. One way is commonly called *scope creep*. During the course of a project, the specifications for the proposed system are allowed to grow with no commensurate allowance in time or budget. The other way is that additional unrelated tasks or projects are piled on, stealing resources from the main system project, again with no adjustment to the main project resources or deadline. The challenge in dealing with these add-on requests is maintaining a positive attitude as the requests mount and the pressure increases. This situation is very susceptible to the straw-that-breaks-the-camel's-back reaction. We accept the early requests pleasantly and then start to progressively grow more negative in responding to additional requests. Soon our reputation as a team player starts to suffer.

Again, the first step in a proactive strategy is to have good data and plans. Then, when given an additional request, our response should be, "Sounds like a good idea to me. Let me look at it and get back to you with the impact on . . ." When the negative impacts will affect a third party, not the requester, the response should be, "It looks like your request would delay Jack's project about a week. Why don't the two of you discuss it and let me know what you want me to do." The key to this approach is being positive and responsive, not negative and querulous.

Plan, Plan, and Plan Some More

The eternal lament: "Why spend all this time planning? We never follow the plan anyway." The true value of planning is as much in the process as it is in the product. To paraphrase Kurt Lewin, you really don't understand a process until you start to *plan* it. A good analogy to this is understanding a complex subject. We may think we understand it until the first time we have to teach it to someone else.

Then we discover all the things we really don't understand, and a whole new level of learning occurs.

There is no definite rule as to how much planning should take place, because projects vary so much. However, a good starting point for many projects is to allow at least 30 percent of the total project calendar time and at least 20 percent of the project resources (money and/or manpower) for the planning stage. As we have said before, this is difficult and frustrating for action-oriented people to do. A common reaction to the numbers we have cited is, "We can't afford all that planning." The implicit assumption is that all that planning time is going to be *added* to the "normal" implementation time. The whole point of good planning is that it *saves* more time and resources than it costs.

The following sections present some key thoughts that we and others have discovered in working with various health informatics projects.

Computerized Planning Processes

In the 1990s, every project should be planned and managed using a computerized project management model. For those of us who started using project management tools in the old batch processing days, it is amazing to see the capabilities and ease of use of today's relatively low-priced microcomputer programs. There are a number of reasons why using this computerized approach is critical.

- Using a formal computerized planning model enforces discipline upon the planner(s). The computer does not respond well to, "You know what I mean." Even if numerous assumptions must be made, a disciplined model forces us to make decisions and choices and often points out illogical or impossible aspects in our plans.
- A computerized model allows easy sensitivity or "what if?" analysis. Manual planning is such tedious work that as soon as a feasible solution is achieved, the planner typically stops, not even making a pretense of searching for optimality. A computerized model allows us to easily test the impact of various strategies or various assumptions, searching for better paths.
- A computerized model allows easy updating and revising of our plans. One of the axioms of planning is, "No battle plan ever survives contact with the enemy." A major shortcoming of manual planning processes is the inconvenience or difficulty in updating those manual plans. The upshot is that

manual plans typically don't get updated often enough, if at all. This means that the management of the project gradually reverts to a continuous ad hoc juggling act.

♦ A computerized model provides tools for easy communication with our various constituencies. The graphical outputs such as Gantt charts are effective in illustrating various points that need to be made. This is also true for other graphical tools such as flow charts or data flow diagrams. The cliché of a picture being worth a thousand words can be very true in communicating complex issues to people who are amateurs or semiprofessionals at best in the project area.

♦ Whether or not using a computerized model truly makes us more organized, it tends to make us look more organized, and that is important. This is not an argument for form over function. The point is that if we are going to be organized, we ought to *project the image* of being organized. It is just one more part of the total marketing effort that all of us must make to operate effectively within an organization.

Plans as Forecasts

Plans are forecasts. This is one of the most misunderstood and abused aspects of planning and the use of plans. Let's look at an example. Suppose that we wish to drive from New York to Los Angeles in February. We might start by selecting a route, taking into account such variables as required arrival date, probable weather, location of friends or relatives with whom we can stay free along the way, sites or attractions we might want to visit along the way, the scenery along various routes, etc. Based upon the route, we then create our time and cost estimates, allowing for at least some unexpected happenings such as weather conditions or minor car problems. We can create a detailed day-by-day plan of costs, mileage, driving hours, places to stay overnight, etc.

What are the chances that our trip will *precisely* follow all the details of our plan? Probably close to zero. What was the advantage of all that planning? It probably enabled us to forestall some potential problems such as not having warm-enough clothes, not having enough money, or not having the car properly prepared. Let's assume that we arrive in Los Angeles on time. Did we still have to make adjustments in our day-to-day plans? We probably did as various events occurred.

More important, with all our planning, could we still miss our arrival deadline? Certainly. Perhaps we encountered the snowstorm of the decade and were snowed in for a week. This means that we have to revise our plan. If our deadline is virtually sacred, we might abandon our car and fly to Los Angeles at a significant increase in cost. If costs are the primary concern, we may spend the snowstorm huddled in our car, surviving on bread and water. There are all kinds of alternatives.

Let's look at a practical basic model that serves very well if it is followed closely. Every project has an *objective*, and it is important to know what the objective is and is not. The objective is *not* the project deadline. It is *not* the project budget. It is *not* the project scope (the system to be implemented). The project objective is to implement that system by that deadline with that budget. If any one of the three is changed, the project objective has been changed. All project objectives and plans are forecasts and are made under a set of assumptions. The formal term for this is *ceteris paribus,* meaning all things equal. Many of these assumptions may be implicit; we assume there will not be a major earthquake, but one can happen. We assume that our highly reputable vendor will not fail us, but it can happen. When the major assumptions do change, we first look at the plan, attempting to make adjustments to compensate. If these adjustments are not enough, the objective must be changed. Which component—the deadline, the budget, the scope, some combination? The right decision is situation-specific.

Apply this model to our travel example. The project objective is to reach Los Angeles (scope) by a certain time (deadline) for a certain cost outlay (budget). As minor problems occur, we juggle resources to adjust, such as driving longer for a day or so, to make up for a day that we were delayed by unforeseen road construction. However, the very bad snowstorm is another matter. There is no juggling of resources that will cover this magnitude of change; therefore; the objective must be changed. Remember, if we fly and get there on time, the objective has still changed because the budget has changed.

If we seem to be overemphasizing this issue, rest assured we are not. The failure to keep these concepts separate is a major cause of miscommunications and recriminations on major projects. This brings us to one final point. All of this refers to significant projects, realizing that the definition of significant can vary widely from person to person or organization to organization. Traveling from New York to Los Angeles is one thing; a trip across town is another in terms of the necessary level of planning and preparation.

Adaptive Planning

In this era of rapid changes, there is a tremendous benefit to creating more *adaptive* plans. In practical terms, that plan is most adaptive that allows irrevocable significant decisions to be made the latest. This is an elaborate way of saying, "Keep options open as long as possible." It is very possible that a price will be paid for this flexibility. For example, if we make this equipment decision right now, we can get a price break that supposedly will not be available later. We view the higher cost of maintaining flexibility as a form of insurance cost—in this case insuring against relevant changes.

Some people express this same basic concept in another way. They argue that in a dynamic area such as today's health informatics arena, detailed planning is difficult or even impossible. They use the term *positioning* to describe the act of maintaining flexibility to cope with future changes. The important issue is the concept, not the exact method or jargon.

Building a Complete Project Plan

Normally, the behavioral acceptance of a new technology is just as important as the actual capabilities of that new technology. Committed people can make weak systems work at least reasonably well; look how they have done it for years! Uncommitted people can easily make a technically superior system work poorly at best. Unfortunately, managers usually focus their efforts and resources on the "concrete" aspects of the new system—its technology and the very basic training of people to use it. They focus few if any resources and efforts on effectively managing the smooth introduction of the technology and systems into the organization.

At the 1993 International Medical Informatics Association (IMIA) Working Conference on the Organizational Impact of Medical Informatics[9] held in Cincinnati, Ohio, a quite experienced information systems manager said to us, "Over the years, I've drawn up a lot of technical plans, but I have never drawn up an organizational one." He went on to say that his future project plans were going to be a lot different. The exact planning structure is not important. We could draw up project plans with a strong *organizational component*. We could draw up a traditional project plan and a separate but coordinated *organizational plan*. Regardless of the jargon used, the point is the same. We need to consciously create a plan for the organizational elements of our implementation process in just the same way that we plan our organizational elements.

Use Team Approaches

In many technical areas, the traditional development process has been a *linear hand-off* model. This means that each major step is performed by a particular group that in turn passes its output to the next group in the sequence. Systems analysis might pass it on to programming, which passes it on to quality assurance, which passes it on to operations. Each group has low ownership in the product once it has moved on and semi-adversarial relationships often develop between the groups. Those upstream often look down on those downstream, and those downstream often shirk responsibility by blaming all problems on those upstream. This is not exactly a team approach. Another problem is that this model is not conducive to involving other stakeholders such as end users in the process.

A more effective approach is the team-oriented *concurrent* model, widely used today in the engineering area. In this model, all the key stakeholders participate in the process from beginning to end, although the intensity of participation may vary over time according to the specific activities of the moment. Quality is not an afterthought. End-user concerns are addressed from the beginning. These are the types of benefits that accrue from this process. Also, total project times are often reduced. The cost is cultural change.

In describing their most effective information systems implementation, Thomas Fischer, the Vice President for Information Management at Kaiser Permanente, described the project as follows:

- the project was staffed with good quality information systems people,
- the information systems people were full time on the project for the most part,
- the end-user area assigned good people to work on the team,
- the information systems people were housed in the end-user area for the duration of the project.[9]

All of these conditions are conducive to the creation of a quality team that, in turn, produced a quality product.

Build Flexible Systems

Those of us who were around in the electronic–dinosaur age remember when the entire economic structure of information systems was completely different. Relatively speaking, computer resources were very expensive and people—both systems developers and end users—were cheap. Therefore, the emphasis was on optimizing the utilization of the "scarce" resource, the computer. Twenty-five years ago, for example, adding 256K (kilobytes) of memory to a mainframe computer cost so much that it was a decision that required board of directors approval. Today, we add a megabyte of memory, four times as much, to our microcomputers for under fifty dollars.

Because of these early economic relationships, a tradition grew of using systems design and programming techniques that would optimize the utilization of this expensive resource, the machine. The needs of the end users were consistently ignored or sacrificed to this optimization process. A culture developed in which the prize programmers were those who could get the most out of the machine, not those who could best meet the users' needs. In addition, the early software tools were primitive by today's standards and produced rigid systems that were difficult to modify, update, and maintain. Acceptance of these limitations also became part of this early culture.

Since those early days, the economic relationships have steadily changed with explosive changes coming over the last decade. Today, computers of all sizes are practically commodity products, while people are the expensive and precious resources. However, the changes in the information systems culture have often not kept up with the changes in economics. We still have many in the information systems field who are heavily influenced by the traditional cultural values.

The pace of change in today's organizations requires that our systems be developed with maximum flexibility in mind. This means the ability to make rapid alterations in the system to accommodate routine updates, changes in load factors, changes in necessary features, the use of new supporting technologies, etc. The price typically paid for this flexibility is twofold. First, it requires substantial amounts of thought and planning early in the systems development process, including significant amounts of interaction with the end users of the system. Second, it tends to produce systems that are relatively inefficient judged by traditional standards of efficiency. Regarding the former, heavy interaction with the end users is one of the core messages of this book and is stressed repeatedly. Regarding the latter, the realities of modern information systems economics have to be addressed. All things equal, efficient systems are more desirable than inefficient systems. However, in this case, all things are not equal. The modern strategy for most situations is to use those tools and approaches that offer the most downstream flexibility and overwhelm any inefficiencies with raw machine power. This is not an "elegant" approach, and it tends to offend the computer purists. However, it is an approach aimed at maximizing the welfare of the end users and the organization, even if it fails to meet the psychic needs of the techies. This is the reality of the modern computer era.

Manage the Key Project Values Well

There are several values issues that need to be well managed on significant projects. These issues fall into two categories: basic project tradeoffs and key project values.

Basic Project Tradeoffs

As discussed earlier, every project objective has three components: deadline, budget, and scope. When consulting on projects, we often ask the project team members and other key stakeholders to give us their individual opinions as to the priority order of these three variables for the particular project. We specify that we are talking about what they *are*, not what they should be. The spread in responses is amazing. Why don't organizations communicate these priorities clearly?

What is the implication of these discrepancies? Why do they exist? Many organizations, especially those with traditional cultures, don't want to give the project team members the impression that they really have any latitude in implementing project priorities. When asked which of the three objective components is the most critical, managers in these organizations respond that all three are important. The problem is that micro-tradeoffs between these three components start on day one of the project implementation. Do we spend another hour polishing this piece of work or do we move on to the next piece? Whether management realizes it or not, this kind of micro-tradeoff is constantly made by team members. If management won't set the priorities for them, the team members will either try to guess what management wants or use their own priorities. The latter is especially true with techies whose priorities are often not parallel with those of the organization. Without clear communication, portions of the team can be making their tradeoffs in conflicting manners.

Key Project Values

Key project values are those one or two values that become the guiding principles by which the project is managed and implemented. For example, a project might have a key value of end-user satisfaction or system flexibility or system reliability (as in the case of a mission-critical clinical operating room system). Again, if these values are not defined and communicated, the constant tradeoffs will be made in a haphazard way.

The six-step process shown below, called "Management by Values," was developed by Riley Associates,[7] and it represents the thinking of many of today's management gurus.

1. The key person or persons must first define and then prioritize the critical values for the project.
2. The values and priorities defined above must be packaged for effective communication to the relevant audience.
3. The values and priorities must be communicated repeatedly with management constantly seeking new examples and ways of expression.
4. The manager(s) must consistently act as role models.
5. Adherence to and support of the values and priorities must be incorporated into the reward structure (in the total sense) and consistently reinforced both positively and negatively.
6. In the absence of negative information, the people must be presumed to be following the values and priorities; that is, they must be trusted.

This type of process can be used on either an individual large project or on a continuous basis within a project-oriented environment.

Constantly Improve Your Management Processes

Achieving successful health informatics implementations requires quality management. A ten-question managerial checklist created by Riley Associates[7] appears below. No set of ten questions can ever completely measure the quality of management; however, this set of questions has been used by thousands of people as an aid to self-assessment and self-improvement in the management area. In this managerial checklist, the word *organization* is used generically and can apply to an entire organization, a department, or a project team.

We always urge people to answer the questions for their own management practices in their own organizations, seeking to identify the most productive areas on which to focus their self-improvement efforts. We urge them also to put a note in their time planners to answer these questions again three months and six months later.

The questions are obvious, "How am I doing? Am I moving in the right direction or not?" When responding to the managerial checklist, select Y (Yes) when the statements clearly apply to your organization; N (No) when the statements clearly do not apply; and the intermediate columns such as Y/N (Yes/No) when things are between. The desirable answers are toward the "Yes" end of the spectrum. If you have the courage, you might ask those you manage to fill out a copy, giving their opinions of how you manage. This can be very revealing.

	Y	Y/N		N
1. An organization must develop and communicate a clear, concise sense of its theme, mission, or direction to all levels of the organization, not just to the top levels. To do this the organization must communicate the "big picture" plus the clear goals and objectives, and at the same time set clear, explicit performance expectations for achieving these directions.	☐	☐	☐	☐	☐
2. An organization must create a strong sense of excitement about the organization and its future development and direction. If the top leadership of an organization is isolated from the lower levels, then it is difficult for the lower levels to have a sense of excitement. The organizational leadership must provide challenges and opportunities for growth at all levels of the organization.	☐	☐	☐	☐	☐
3. An organization must build a sense of ownership and participation at all levels. A truly successful organization will reduce or eliminate unilateral top-down decision making. Managers will solicit and heed quality inputs from employees at all levels. They will adequately communicate the "Why" of decisions, and they will frequently delegate tasks rather than assign them. They will work diligently to avoid developing a caste system.	☐	☐	☐	☐	☐

4. A successful organization will invest high energy in the staffing process at all levels. Managers will accurately define the real success characteristics within the organization. They will have an ever-expanding recruiting pool for future employees. Widespread participation in the employee selection process will be encouraged. Finally, the successful organization will have an intensive orientation process for new employees to help implant the desired organizational values.

5. The successful organization will provide adequate rewards and support to the staff and will utilize the "human capital" concept to encourage and nurture their employees. The successful organization will recognize the important of all team members and will balance the monetary and psychic rewards for everyone, not just a chosen few.

6. The successful organization moves fast to halt poor performance by anyone at any level of the organization. There are high standards of performance and ways to distinguish incompetence or "attitudinal" errors from reasonable "growth" errors. Management is willing to pay a heavy price, if necessary, to remove those who deliberately perform at substandard levels.

7. The successful organization provides an atmosphere of trust and integrity for all the employees. There is a uniform and impartial system for the distribution of rewards and discipline. There is truthfulness in both formal and informal communications. Managers precisely define and subsequently fulfill completely all their promises. They do not subject employees to intricate and/or humiliating internal control systems, which indicates low levels of trust .

8. The successful organization provides a ☐ ☐ ☐ ☐ ☐
stable organizational environment for the
employees. It does not subject the employees
to frequent hasty reactive decisions that
subsequently have to be changed. There is a
stable organizational structure that works
effectively. Management does not force
employees to develop numerous informal
systems to make an inadequate formal system
actually work.

9. The successful organization maintains ☐ ☐ ☐ ☐ ☐
accurate and timely two-way communication
with staff and customers—both internal and
external. It pursues feedback from both
satisfied and unsatisfied customers and staff.
It establishes a climate in which staff
members at all levels feel free to communicate
their concerns. The organization periodically
reinforces and/or updates communications
that are of continuing relevance.

10. The successful organizational environment ☐ ☐ ☐ ☐ ☐
encourages and supports risk taking and
entrepreneurship by employees at all levels. It
encourages, supports, and rewards constantly
the development of new systems and the
improvement of old ones. Managers allow
reasonable "learning" errors and coach for the
potential subordinate growth and development that could result from these errors. They
encourage and even demand a reasonable
level of staff independence.

Conclusion

As we come to the end of our discussion on project management, let
us review another anonymous piece of tongue-in-cheek photocopier
graffiti that is usually entitled the "Laws of Project Management" or
something similar. Like all such, it is grossly exaggerated for
emphasis; however, if there were no truth in it, it would never have
been written, and we would not chuckle as we read it. Review these
eight "laws" carefully and contrast them with your experiences.

1. No major informatics project is ever installed on time, within budget, and with the same staff that started it. Yours will not be the first.

2. A carelessly planned project will take three times longer than expected to complete; a carefully planned project will only take twice as long.

3. A major advantage of fuzzy project objectives is that they let you avoid the embarrassment of accurately estimating their costs.

4. When the project is going well, something will go wrong. When things can't get worse, they will. When things appear to be going better, you have overlooked something.

5. Informatics project teams detest progress reporting because it clearly exposes their lack of progress.

6. If the scope of an informatics project is allowed to change freely, the rate of change will far exceed the rate of progress.

7. Major informatics projects progress quickly until they are 90 percent complete and then remain 90 percent complete forever.

8. No major informatics system is ever completely debugged, and efforts to debug the system inevitably produce new bugs that are even harder to find.

In this chapter, we have presented some crucial aspects of quality project planning and management approaches to the implementation of health informatics systems. Those unfamiliar with basic project management principles and practices should seek additional help in this critical area, as good project planning and management are essential to systems implementation. One of the aspects that must be planned for is the management of the organizational change that will be produced by the implementation. The next chapter will focus on these concepts and practices of sound change management.

Questions

1. What benefits might intensive planning efforts reap beside those presented in this chapter?
2. Describe the following clearly in your own words: the project objective, the project scope, the project budget, the project deadline, and the project plan.
3. After reviewing the managerial checklist presented in this chapter, how would you rank the ten question areas in their order of importance in ensuring good management? Would your answers vary according to the level of management? To the functional area being managed?
4. In terms of estimating completion times, do you see yourself as an optimist, pessimist, or realist? Why? If an optimist or pessimist, what prices do you pay?
5. Describe a situation you have personally observed in which the parties failed to resolve conflicts early in the relationship or process. What prices did the parties later pay for their failure?

References

1.   Meredith, JR, Mantel, SJ Jr. *Project Management: A Managerial Approach,* second edition. New York: John Wiley & Sons, 1989.
2.   Kidder, T. *The Soul of a New Machine.* New York: Avon Books, 1981.
3.   Currid, C. A case against CASE: It's expensive and often unsuccessful. *Infoworld* August 2, 1993;68.
4.   Power, C. et al. Flops: Too many new products fail. Here's why-and how to do better. *Business Week* August 16, 1993;76–82.
5.   Getting smart about new products: How a company can improve its success rate in product launches. *Business Week* August 16, 1993;78–79.
6.   Trachtenberg, JA. Interactive kiosks may be high-tech but they underwhelm US. consumers. *Wall Street Journal* March 14, 1994;B1–B8.
7.   Riley, RT. *The Engineer as Manager.* Cincinnati: Riley Associates, 1987.
8.   Horak, B. Implementation-time productivity. *Organizational Issues in Medical Informatics* 1993;October:1–2.
9.   *Draft Proceedings of the International Medical Informatics Association Working Conference on the Organizational Impact of Informatics.* Cincinnati: Riley Associates, 1993.

8
Change Management for Successful Implementation

> Its exciting to think about a new vision particularly when you're the creator/driver of it. You see the need clearly. You feel the urgency in your stomach. You're motivated to change. You see the fire with your own eyes. Your smell the smoke in your own nostrils. The tent is on fire. You have to change. Why are others in the organization so lackadaisi- cal? Don't they smell the smoke? Don't they see the fire? Don't they feel the urgency to change?[1]

The rate of change in virtually all organizations is escalating, and health care organizations—after a slow start—are no exception. However, this change is often not so exciting when you are on the receiving end. In fact, these changes may be downright threatening to many. Therefore, the phrase *change management* has become fairly common, appearing in management articles everywhere. Review the job ads in the *Wall Street Journal* or the Sunday edition of a major newspaper and notice the positions available for people skilled in change management.

What is change management? What is a "change agent" or a change management person? How does change management help people feel less threatened? How did it evolve, and why does everyone seem so fixated on it today? One reason for this fixation is a realization of the tremendous "hidden" costs involved in many informatics implementations. According to the *Wall Street Journal*, "Indeed analysts estimate that the 'true' cost of a PC—including installing it, maintaining it, training people to use it and updating it if necessary—could approach $40,000 over five years or more than 10 times the cost of a high-end machine."[2] The initial cost of a system may be only the tip of the proverbial iceburg when implementing systems—even when the implementation is successful. Unless changes are managed well, the people costs, many of which are buried in other budgets, can skyrocket and dwarf the supposed cost of the system.

What is Change Management?

The health care industry and other businesses as well are constantly trying to reassess their future direction. Some organizations seemed to go through a series of management "fads" in their search for some sort of organizational nirvana. For example, one past fad was Management by Objectives (MBO), an excellent concept for certain organizations at certain stages of organizational growth. Many organizations seized upon it as a cure-all and proceeded to implement it poorly. While proclaiming that they had adopted an MBO philosophy, they actually only paid "lip-service" to the concept. Many people in these organizations were performing rituals such as completing objectives forms, while little actually changed in their daily work lives.

Total Quality Management (TQM) and Continuous Quality Improvement (CQI) are systems that many organizations have adopted today. Most of these implementations are faring no better than MBO did. Rather than truly working to change the organizational culture, many of the adopters have simply installed a new set of rituals. Rather than leading the effort for change, top management delegates the process to staff and gallops off to deal with crises in the same old way. The danger is that this concept called change management may meet the same fate.

Change management is the process by which an organization gets to its future state—the vision. Traditional planning processes delineate the steps on the journey. The role of change management is to facilitate that journey. Therefore, creating change starts with creating a vision for change and then empowering individuals to act as change agents to attain that vision. The empowered change management agents need plans that are (1) a total systems approach, (2) realistic, and (3) future oriented. Change management encompasses the effective strategies and programs to enable the champions to achieve the new vision.

This chapter looks at the antecedents of change management, including theories of change and theories in the social sciences. It also presents a proven model for designing strategies for an effective change management process.

Early Change Theory

In 1974, Watzlawick, Weakland, and Fisch published their now classic book, *Change: Principles of Problem Formation and Problem Resolution*.[3] Theories about change had long existed. However,

Watzlawick et al. found that most of the theories of change were philosophical and derived from the areas of mathematics and physics. Watzlawick and his coauthors selected two theories from the field of mathematical logic upon which to base their beliefs about change. They selected the theory of groups and the theory of logical types. Their goal of reviewing the theories of change was to explain the accelerated phenomenon of change that they were witnessing. Let's briefly look at the two theories that Watzlawick et al. reviewed to develop their change theory.

The more sophisticated implications of the *theory of groups* can be appreciated only by mathematicians or physicists. Its basic postulates concern the relationships between parts and wholes. According to the theory, a group has several properties, including members that are all alike in one common characteristic. These members can be numbers, objects, concepts, events, or whatever else one wants to draw together in such a group, as long as they have at least one common denominator. Another property of a group is the ability to combine the members of the group in a number of varying sequences and have the same combinations. The theory of groups gives a model for the types of change that transcend a given system.

The *theory of logical types* begins with the concept of collections of "things" that are united by a specific characteristic common to all of them. For example, mankind is the name for all individuals, but mankind is not a specific individual. Any attempt to change one in terms of the other does not work and leads to nonsense and confusion. For example, the economic behavior of the population of a large city cannot be understood in terms of the behavior of one person multiplied by four million. A population of four million people is not just quantitatively but also qualitatively different from an individual. Similarly, while the individual members of a species are usually endowed with very specific survival mechanisms, the entire species may race headlong toward extinction—and the human species is probably no exception.

The theory of groups gave Watzlawick's group the framework for thinking about the kind of change that can occur within a system that itself stays invariant. The theory of logical types is not concerned with what goes on inside a class, but gave the authors a framework for considering the relationship between member and class and the peculiar metamorphosis that is in the nature of shifts from one logical level to the next higher. From this, they concluded that there are two different types of change: one that occurs within a given system that itself remains unchanged, and one whose occurrence changes the system itself. For example, a person having a nightmare can do many things in his dream—hide, fight, scream, jump off a cliff, etc. But no change from any one of these behaviors to another would terminate the nightmare. Watzlawick et al. concluded that this is a first-order change. The one way out of a dream involves a change from dreaming to waking. Waking is no longer a part of the dream, but a change to an altogether different state. This is their second-order change as outlined in Chapter 2. When the Watzlawick book was published, many people were unfamiliar with the applications of theories of change into contemporary society; thus, the book was a major contribution for alternative ways of looking at the changes that occur daily.

Change Management Psychology

While Watzlawick et al. comprehensively presented the theories of change and offered their model of levels of change, they did not offer practical day-to-day strategies. We are interested in the effective strategies for managing change and have reviewed many social science theories to determine the psychology behind the change management concepts and strategies that are used widely today. We believe that today's successful change management strategies emanate from several theories in the areas of psychology and sociology. Small group theories and field theories provide the antecedents of today's successful change management practices.

Small Group Theories

The *primary group* is one of the classical concepts of sociology, and many sociological theories focus on small-group analysis and the interaction process analysis. These theories outline and delineate small-group behavior. Small-group theories help us to understand not only how to make things more successful, but also how to analyze when things go wrong. One practical application of small-group research was presented by Bales in the *Harvard Business Review*.[4] Bales applies small group principles to running a meeting, and makes the following suggestions:

- If possible, restrict committees to seven members.
- Place all members so they can readily communicate with every other member.
- Avoid committees as small as two or three if a perceived power problem between members is likely to be critical.

- ◆ Select committee members who are likely to participate in varying amounts. A group with all highly active participants or all low participants will be difficult to manage.

We have all seen small-group behavior at work. For example, a job candidate is interviewed by a number of people. Information is then collected from the interviewers and is shared with a search committee. The search committee selects their top candidate, and that person is hired. If the person hired does not work out, a member of the search committee may very well say, "I knew that Mary would not work out, but I didn't say anything because everyone seemed to like her."

Many of the changes that new technology brings are discussed, reviewed, debated by groups of people that usually fall within the small-group framework. If negative sentiments about a product or service are stated by a member of the group who is an opinion leader, the less-vocal people will often not challenge the dominant opinion. For example, a medium-sized organization was selecting a local area network (LAN) system. While the senior leader wanted one system, some of the other people not only had suggestions, but documentation of the qualities of another system. During the meeting to decide which system to purchase, the senior leader stated his views first and quite strongly. A couple of the lower-level staff members started to confront the senior person; however, when there was no support from any of the other people present, they did not express their strong preferences for their system of choice. When the system finally arrived, the senior leader's initial enthusiasm had dwindled. He then confronted the technology people as to why they had not made him aware of the shortcomings of the system selected.

These examples lead us to a change management principle: to effectively manage change, it is imperative for change agents to understand how people behave in groups and especially in small groups.

Field Theory

Kurt Lewin and his students are credited with combining theories from psychology and sociology into the field theory in social psychology.[5] Lewin focused his attention on motivation and the motivational concepts that underlie an individual's behavior. Lewin believed that there is tension within a person whenever a psychological need or an intention exists, and the tension is released only when the need or intention is fulfilled. The tension may be positive or negative. These positive and negative tension concepts were translated into a more refined understanding of conflict situations and, in turn, what Lewin called "force fields."

Lewin indicated that there are three fundamental types of conflict:

1. The individual stands midway between two positive goals of approximately equal strength. A classic metaphor is the donkey starving between two stacks of hay because of the inability to choose. In information technology, if there are two "good" systems to purchase or options to pursue, then we must be willing to choose.

2. The individuals find themselves between two approximately equal negative goals. This certainly has been a conflict within many organizations wishing to purchase or build a health informatics systems. A combination of the economics, the available technologies, the organizational issues, etc., may well mean that the organization's informatics needs cannot be satisfied with any of the available products—whether purchased or developed in-house. Thus the decision makers must make a choice of an information system that they know will not completely meet their needs. Their choice will probably be the lesser of two evils.

3. The individual is exposed to opposing positive and negative forces. This conflict is very common in health care organizations today, especially regarding health informatics. This conflict usually occurs between the systems users and the information technology people or the financial people.

    For example, one hospital decided to implement a new computer system for its clinical laboratory. The hospital CEO decided on the maximum price for the system before the planners began calculating system capabilities to meet user needs. The clinical laboratory was a very complex and busy organization. Therefore, when the needs were fully outlined, the basic hardware and software were more costly than originally budgeted by the CEO. Faced with the positive (an automated laboratory system) and the negative (an under-powered system because of finances) the members of the planning group and the CIO recommended purchasing a smaller than needed laboratory system. As soon as the system was operational, everyone was understandably "upset" with it. The system did not meet the needs of the clinical laboratory, it did not meet the needs of the physicians and nurses, and ultimately, it did not meet the needs of the total organization. The CEO blamed the head of the clinical laboratory, and eventually that person was replaced. We wonder to this day if that CEO ever realized his role in the creation of this disaster.

Another type of positive-negative conflict occurs frequently between a clinical system's end users and the needs of the total organization. In one hospital, representatives from an obstetrics department did extensive research on the type of clinical information system that would best meet the needs of their patients, especially since their patients visit clinicians before, during, and after the birth of the child. Based upon this research, they selected a system (positive force) and then presented their decision to their parent organization's CIO. The information technology people could not decide if the system desired by the obstetrics professionals would blend into the system that they were designing for the total hospital. Therefore, instead of saying yes or no, the CIO said nothing (negative force), which greatly increased stress levels within the organization.

All of these social science theories assist the change management leader in understanding some of the underlying behavior issues as they bring health informatics technology into today's complex health systems.

What Do These Theories Mean to Change Management?

People can easily be overwhelmed by change, especially within large organizations where they may perceive they have little or no voice in or control over the changes they perceive are descending upon them. The typical response is fight or flight, not cooperation. Managers often interpret such human resistance to change as "stubbornness" or "not being on the team." This reaction solves nothing in terms of reducing resistance to change or gaining acceptance of it. Many managers do not accept that they are regarded as imposing "life-threatening" changes and establishing "no-win" adversary relationships between management and those below in the organization.

Small-group theory is highly applicable because of the way that medical environments are organized. The care of the patient or the education of students entails many small groups. These groups converse and share information and feelings, and strong opinion leaders can sway others to their way of thinking relatively easily.

Kurt Lewin's field theory allows the diagramming of the types of conflict situations commonly found in health care. A practical illustration of Kurt Lewin's original force field approach is shown in Table 8.1. We have used some of the typical resistance examples, originally raised in Chapter 2.

There are several critical points in this force-field diagram:

◆   Every change, whether actual or proposed, is characterized primarily by the goal or termination point intended as a result of the change. The goal is often multiple and in series, such as a change intended to (1) implement a new information system in order to (2) improve patient care.

← Negative Forces	Positive Forces →
Whose idea was this? Nobody asked me. ◄———	
	More efficiency (cut labor costs). ———►
I have my own way and I like it fine, thank you. ◄———	
	Better patient care. ———►
Will we lose our jobs? ◄———	
	Reclassifications and more money. ———►
I like the people I work with. I don't want to work with new people. ◄———	
	New status for staff. ———►
Why didn't they give us some decent training? ◄———	

Table 8.1. Force field analysis of some of the typical change resistance comments.

- Every change creates effects upon people and existing systems, some intended and some unintended, i.e., side effects.
- In most change processes, the forces operating will be either positive (moving people to accept and cooperate with the change) or negative (driving people to resist, fight, and work against either the change or its manner of implementation). These forces vary from "strong" to "weak" as represented in the diagram by the length of the arrow.
- Forces in the diagram are either real or imagined. For example, a negative force in a particular situation, might be "fear of facing retraining" which, in fact, is real—the change will require extensive retraining. But another negative force might be "fear of layoff" which, in fact, is mere rumor and imaginary; however, these negative forces remain in effect, whether real or imagined, so long as people perceive they might be true.

The conflicts of approach-avoidance that Lewin discusses are prevalent. For example, if I accept this new system, what will it mean to me and my job? Will I have a job? How will it change my role? Will this new system lessen my role? The anxieties expressed by these questions are very clear and very real to the people within the system. Remember what we said in Chapter 2: one person's microchanges are often another person's megachanges. So as the system designers think they are making a minor change to enhance the total system, an individual end user may see the change as a megachange and resist it vehemently.

When designing the total "people" strategy for any system, it is important to involve the people from the very beginning and to clearly understand how groups function within the organization.

Change Management Strategies

Change management is the process of assisting individuals and organizations of passing from an old way of doing things to a new way of doing things. A change process should both begin and end with a visible acknowledgment or celebration of the impending or just completed change. James Belasco says,

Our culture is filled with empowering transitions. New Year's Eve parties symbolize the ending of one year and the hope to be found in the one just beginning. Funerals are times to remember the good points of the loved one and the hope for new beginnings elsewhere.

Parties given to retiring or leaving employees are celebrations of the ending of the employee's past status and the hope for the new opportunities to be found in the new status."1

Based on our research, there is not one change management strategy that can be used in every situation. It is essential for the change management leader to take the time to know the desired state (vision-goal) and the particular organization and then to develop the appropriate strategies and plans to help facilitate the desired state.

Over the years we have evolved a core model for the major process of change management. There are many options within this model, but we believe that it is helpful for leaders to have an overview map in mind as they begin to implement new information technology systems. The five-stage model that has proven effective for reducing barriers to technology change begins with an assessment and information-gathering phase.6

Assessment

The assessment phase of this model is the foundation for determining the organizational and user knowledge and ownership of the health informatics system that is under consideration. Ideally this phase of the model begins even before the planning for the technological implementation of the new system. The longer the delay, the harder it will be to successfully manage the change and gain ultimate user ownership.

There are two parts to the assessment phase. The first is to *inform* all potentially affected people, in writing, of the impending change. This written information need not be lengthy or elaborate, but it will alert everyone to the changes in process.

The second part involves *collecting information* from those involved in the change by the use of both surveys and interviews. The survey instrument should be sent to randomly selected members of the affected group. One person in ten might be appropriate if the affected group is large. Five to ten open-ended questions should assess the individuals' current perceptions of the potential changes, their issues of greatest concern about these changes, and their suggestions to reduce those concerns. Recording and analyzing the responders' demographics will allow more in-depth analysis of the concerns raised by these potentially affected people.

In the personal face-to-face interviews with randomly selected people at all levels throughout the affected portions of the organization, it is important to listen to the stories the people are telling and to assess their positive and negative feelings about the proposed health informatics system. These interviews should help in ascertaining the current levels of positive and negative feelings; what each person envisions the future will be, both with and without the new system; what each interviewee could contribute to making that vision a reality; and how the interviewee could contribute to the future success of the new system. These interviews provide critical insights for the actual implementation plan. Often those people interviewed become advocates—and sometimes even champions—of the new system, thus easing the change process considerably.

An alternative or supplement to the one-on-one interviews is focus-group sessions. These allow anywhere from five to seven people from across the organization to share their feelings and ideas about the current system and new system.

Feedback and Options

The information obtained above must now be analyzed, integrated, and packaged for presentation to both top management and to those directly responsible for the technical implementation. This is a key stage for understanding the strengths and weaknesses of the current plans, identifying the major organizational areas of both excitement and resistance (positive and negative forces), identifying the potential stumbling blocks, understanding the vision the staff holds for the future, and reviewing the options suggested by the staff for making the vision come true. If this stage occurs early enough in the process, data from the assessment stage can be given to the new system developers for review.

When designing your model, this phase is important in order to establish that the organization *learns* from the inputs of its staff and begins to act strategically in the decision and implementation processes.

Strategy Development

This phase of the model allows those responsible for the change to use the information collected to develop *effective change strategies* from an organizational perspective. These strategies must focus on a visible, effective process to "bring on board" the affected people within the organization. This could include newsletters, focus groups, discussions, one-on-one training, and confidential "hand-holding." This latter can be especially important for professionals such as physicians who may not wish to admit ignorance and/or apprehension about the new system.

Implementation

This phase of our model refers to the implementation of the change management strategies determined to be needed for the organization, not to the implementation of the new system. The implementation of the change strategies developed above must begin before the actual implementation of the new system. These behaviorally focused efforts consist of a series of steps, including informing and working with the people involved in a systematic and timely manner. This step-by-step progression toward the behavioral change desired and the future goals is important to each individual's acceptance of the new system. This is an effective mechanism for tying together the new technology implementation action plan with the behavioral strategies.

Reassessment

Six months after the new system is installed, a behavioral-effects data-gathering process should be conducted. This stage resembles the initial assessment stage—written surveys and one-on-one and/or focus-group interviews. Data gathered from this stage allow measurement of the acceptance of the new system, which provides the basis for fine-tuning. This process also serves as input to the evaluation of the implementation process. It assures all the participants that their inputs and concerns are still valued and sought, even though the particular implementation has already occurred.

Conclusion

Change is difficult, but eventually it happens. Successful change stories continue to grow. Some of the change is smooth and some of the change difficult, but nonetheless change is happening.

It is not always easy to know exactly why a particular group resists change. However, experience shows that an intelligent application of this basic five-step change model—coupled with a sound technological implementation plan—leads to more rapid and more productive introductions of technology into organizations. The process can be expensive in terms of time and energy but nowhere near the cost of an expensive technical system that never gains real user acceptance.

Perhaps most important, overall success requires an emotional commitment to success on the part of all involved. The people must believe the project is being done for the right reasons—namely, to further the delivery of higher quality, more cost-effective health care. If a project is generally perceived to be aimed at just "saving a quick buck" or boosting someone's ego or status, that project is doomed to fail.

Questions

1. What is your definition of change management?
2. What are some ways to help people celebrate remembering the past and moving to the future?
3. Complete a force field analysis of an information technology problem you have experienced.
4. Why is the "feedback and options" phase so important in the change management model presented?

References

1. Belasco, JA. *Teaching the Elephant To Dance: Empowering Change in Your Organization.* New York: Crown Publishers, 1990.
2. Pope, K. ComputerLand changes name as part of new focus, gets outsourcing work. *Wall Street Journal* March 22, 1994;B-8.
3. Watzlawick, P, Weakland, JH, Fisch, R. *Change: Principles of Problem Formation and Problem Resolution.* New York: W.W. Norton, 1974.
4. Bales, RF. In conference. *Harvard Business Review* 1954;32:44–50.
5. Deutsch, M, Krauss, RM. *Theories in Social Psychology.* New York: Basic Books, 1965.
6. Lorenzi, NM, Mantel, MI, Riley, RT. Preparing your organizations for technological change. *Healthcare Informatics*, 1990; December:33–34.

9
Negotiating the Political Minefields

A leader of an integrated health care information effort once told us, "I knew our project was necessary and important when suddenly everyone wanted to take it away from me." We have all probably found ourselves in a political quagmire and wondered how we got there. This is especially true when we are "just certain" that we have covered all the bases or we consider ourselves to be a "good politician." One often-expressed concept is that the more widespread use of information technology will stimulate the flow of information and eliminate traditional organizational hierarchies. A possible inference—or desperate hope—is that this will then reduce the amount of politics in the organization. However, more people are now realizing that information and the control of it are still key organizational "currencies."

Whether we like it or not, introducing any type of change into an organization, but especially a technological change, is inevitably a very political process. These political issues surrounding both information and information technology management in information-based organizations must be addressed. We deliberately did not mention the political issues in the last chapter, but they will always consume a major portion of the change leader's energies. Therefore, this chapter is devoted to understanding and negotiating the political minefields.

"Say It Ain't So, Charlie Brown"

Just when you think you are making good progress on your project and have touched all the bases, the infamous "grapevine" starts telling you that you have problems. You are surprised and you wonder what's happening. One senior information systems person said to us that he did not like politics; therefore, he was going to stay out of all the organizational politics and just do his "job." While this may be an attractive fantasy for many of us, in reality a major portion of our jobs is effectively dealing with the organizational political process.

Examples of Political Problems

When we attempt to introduce complex informatics systems, most of the problems fall into the general "Yes, but . . ." category, which is found in such comments as "Great idea, but . . ." "I really support this effort, but . . ." "This is good, but . . ." and "I support you strongly, but . . ." These reactions have a variety of political ramifications and play out in different ways depending upon the political skills of those involved. We have seen all of the following examples occur at least once in various organizations.

"Great Idea, But . . ."

A hospital administrator once said that he really supported the integrated information concept, but he was concerned that the physicians would really like the proposed prototype and would then want the system implemented throughout the hospital, pressuring him to find the money for it. He said that if the project leader could raise all the money from outside sources, then it would be okay with him to implement the prototype. The organizational conflict was between the needs of the clinicians and the willingness of the hospital to support anything but a major financial-based information system. Some of the major stakeholders in this organization had very different objectives, and the change leader was caught in the political crossfire between the groups.

A variation in this category is, "Great idea, but do it my way." In one organization, a new chief executive officer arrived and liked the fact that the organization was moving toward a clinical information system. However, he decided that the information system used in his last hospital was an excellent system and should be transported intact to his new location. Even though many of the clinicians at his new site had different thoughts about what constituted a good clinical information system, the new CEO only wanted the "same system as we had back at my old place."

Another variant occurs when CIOs say, "Great idea, but you are going about this in the wrong way." They then pressure you heavily to use—and pay for, of course—this wonderful new technology that they are desperately trying to fund. It may be a poor choice for your needs.

"I Really Support This Effort, But . . ."

There are a number of endings that go with this "Yes, but . . ." Some examples: "The organization is just not ready for this project." "I don't like the particular technology you have selected." "You didn't include me as much as you should have." "I don't like where you are going to place the terminals." "I don't really think our nurses will have time for this new technology." "I could do it better."

The comments in this category are the sniping type, consisting typically of snide remarks and potshots. Often arising from jealousy, they are attempts to undermine organizational confidence in the project. These comments are typically made to third parties—ideally the big boss—rather than to the implementer. What often makes these especially frustrating to the implementer is that the snipers' opinions may well have been solicited earlier, but the requests were ignored.

"This is Really Good, But . . ."

There are just a couple of endings for this "Yes, but . . ." and they are "But, I want it" and "But, you are going to have to change it." The people in this category are the power players, the Sherman Tanks. They see a project that they could never have started themselves, but, as completion draws closer, they want to take over. They are usually brash, pushy, and opinionated, and they seem to feel they are right about everything or at least convey that image.

In one organization, a physician, who had not been part of the strategic information effort and its subsequent implementation process effort, decided that he had a better idea. He was basically a negative person who found it easier to criticize an effort that he was not leading than to support it. Also, he appeared to be very well informed about information technology issues to those who were not, although certainly not to those who were. This articulate and persuasive person contacted the chief executive officer and made a rather dynamic presentation about his skills and knowledge. At the same time, he made a plea for his inclusion in the process. Rather than saying that there was an established corporate process that was proceeding well, the CEO inserted the physician into the process where he added nothing but wasted immense amounts of the leader's time. Even worse, this was done without consulting with the current leader of the information initiative. The CEO's rationale was that it wouldn't hurt to have more inputs. Incidentally, this physician had no institutional power base other than what the CEO was giving him.

The CEO badly undermined the entire information effort in this case by not involving and supporting the information technology leader. Once installed in the process, the physician used his newfound derived power to continue his aggressive behavior, such as trying to establish a new governing committee parallel to the established one, talking to the technical staff about "his newer and better" model, and talking to some of the hospital staff about problems and issues in the main effort rather than trying to help solve them. The politics in this scenario was highly negative for all concerned and very costly for the organization's information initiative.

"I Support You Fully, But . . ."

Some of the endings here are the following: ". . . but, I have no time right now." ". . . but, you go do it, and I will write a letter of support." ". . . but, you go do it and report back." This is a very dangerous political scenario. The people in this category are always very supportive in face-to-face encounters. They send out letters that you draft for them. In speeches, they say just about anything you want them to say. The problem is they are totally passive in internal political conflicts. They do not want to get involved in any political issues. If problems arise, their "plates" are full; they cannot help out at this moment, but please keep them informed.

In all these scenarios, the political process has become negative; salvaging any semblance of order from these situations is very difficult. The thrust of this chapter is problem prevention, although many of the techniques will at least help in situations that have turned negative. However, there are negative political situations in which the only solution is major personnel changes—major in terms of level or numbers or both.

Politics and Power

Part of our problem with politics may stem from the negative connotation of the word itself. For many of us, the word conjures up images of smoke-filled rooms and underhanded tactics. In many current job-status studies, politics as a profession ranks quite low in status and image. On the other hand, words such as persuading, influencing, inducing, convincing, or negotiating would not cause the same near-revulsion in many of us. However pleasant these euphemisms might be, the reality is that our organizations are political systems, and we may as well address the issues of politics and power directly. Anyone who has read *The Prince* by Machiavelli, written more than 450 years ago, knows that political strategizing has been around for a long time. "Politics is both the cause and the effect of transitional forces exerted by specific areas of interest. As the world continues to change, participation in the political process becomes more imperative."[1]

If you are responsible for a implementing a major health informatics system or other major change in the organization, you must either be a part of the organizational "power structure" or have its strong direct support. If you are not part of the power structure, then you must deliberately find ways to ensure that your knowledge and skills are recognized and accepted by the power structure. You then function as a bridge between the power structure and the rest of the organization with respect to the system you are charged with implementing.

Sources of Power

Various management theoreticians use different taxonomies to describe the sources of power. We use a composite one that we have found useful over the years. The importance of such a taxonomy is that it gives us a tool or thought process for analyzing why Dr. X seems to have so much more power than Dr. Y in our environment even though Dr. Y might supposedly "outrank" Dr. X.

There are several types of power:

*   *Interpersonal power* is the ability of one individual to influence the actions of other individuals, independent of other variables. To use a military example, all second lieutenants are created equal by law; however, one says, "Follow me!" and the troops follow. Another says, "Follow me!" and the troops laugh. Interpersonal power is the difference. The most dramatic example of interpersonal power is the form we call charisma—the ability to overwhelm by force of personality. However, there are many components in organizational life such as the abilities to negotiate, influence, sell, persuade, etc. Also, variables such as perceived bravery, integrity, and morality can affect interpersonal power. In more primitive settings, physical power can be a dramatic source of interpersonal power. A definite danger of interpersonal power is that an effective persuader can be sincerely selling a terrible idea.
*   *Knowledge-expertise power* derives from one's abilities in a recognized skill area—typically a technical one. The skilled

nurse, physician, or systems analyst all have definite power, especially among their professional peers. The danger of expertise power can be the fear of the holder that sharing the expertise will cost the holder power.

◆ *Knowledge-information power* stems from, "I know something you don't; therefore . . ." The information has to be perceived to be of some value for power to accrue. Again, the danger is obvious; hoarding can be seen as a source of power even if it is negative for the organization.

◆ *Positional power* derives from the organizational role or position that one occupies and is often thought of as "formal" power. The organization confers the authority to reward, punish, allocate resources, approve, disapprove, delegate, etc. This form of power is important but is easy to overrate. Remember the second lieutenants. As a general rule, the reflexive willingness of the work force to bow to positional power has declined rapidly in industrialized countries in recent years.

◆ *Derived power* is a form of second-hand power that arises when one person appears to have the ear of, or even the right to speak for, a powerful person. The executive secretary often has high derived power in the eyes of the organization. Similarly, people who are protégés or friends of a power person may be perceived to have derived power whether they seek it or not.

◆ *Referent power* is akin to interpersonal power but operates at more of a distance. This is the "monkey see, monkey do" form of power. Referent power is created when people model their behaviors on the behaviors of someone they admire. To parents' endless dismay, the most dramatic examples occur when teenagers model their dress or language or behaviors on their latest pop-culture idol. Adults in organizations will often do the same, emulating the habits or mannerisms of respected leaders. If a respected boss uses a fountain pen, lots of fountain-pen users spring up in the organization.

Remember several points when you think about the above list. First, the sources are not listed in their order of importance. Their relative importance is highly situational. Second, for power to be effective under realistic organizational circumstances, the power must be *accepted* or even *granted* by those on the receiving end. We can attempt to use our interpersonal power; for it to work, it must be accepted or granted by those others. Finally, if we return to the question of why Dr. X has more power than Dr. Y, there may be a combination of sources of power that explains the situation. For a practical discussion of power including self-diagnostic exercises, we recommend *Executive Survival Manual* by Dennis Slevin.[2]

The "Compleat" Manager

Izaak Walton may have told us all about *The Compleat Angler*, but we need to look for a moment at the concept of the "compleat" manager. In seminars, we often use a silly diagram similar to Figure 9.1 to illustrate a key point. The "person" on the left represents the typical human with what we think of as the standard five senses: the physical abilities to feel, hear, see, smell, and taste. These five senses are very closely linked to "doing" or personally performing lots of tasks. People lacking one or more of these basic senses are often still quite productive on many tasks through the intense development of the other senses to compensate.

However, successful managers and systems implementers face challenges that extend beyond just getting tasks done. Understanding power and politics requires a sensitivity to variables beyond those of our particular technologies. Therefore, the managers and implementers need two more things, the antennae shown on the person on the right in Figure 9.1. Ideally, these antennae are invisible or you will receive strange looks around the office. However, their invisibility makes them no less real. Why two of them, other than to meet the needs of some people for symmetry? One of these antennae should be tuned to receive *emotions and feelings*, the other to receive *values and beliefs*.

What happens to these antennae when we become preoccupied with the task aspects of our jobs? They are turned off or retracted or whatever other metaphor you care to use. People may be sending us numerous subtle messages, cues, hints, etc., and they pass right over our heads unnoticed.

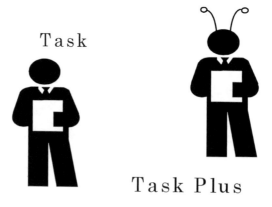

Task

Task Plus

Figure 9.1. The manager's need for antennae.

As we proceed through this and some of the following chapters dealing with both people and organizations, remember that these concepts will not be of much help unless our antennae are turned on and waving in the breeze. It is a definite challenge for many people to move from the task level to the task-plus level as depicted in Figure 9.1.

Swimming Among the Sharks

Writing under the nom de plume of Voltaire Cousteau, Dr. Richard Johns of Johns Hopkins University, evidently an experienced administrator with plenty of scars, wrote a tongue-in-cheek essay entitled, "How to Swim with Sharks: A Primer."[3] Dr. Johns presented this as an essay written for the benefit of French sponge divers by a little known author believed to be a descendant of Voltaire and an ancestor of Jacques Cousteau. Dr. Johns claimed to have translated it from the original French.

> Actually, nobody wants to swim with sharks. It is not an acknowledged sport, and it is neither enjoyable nor exhilarating. These instructions are written primarily for the benefit of those who, by virtue of their occupation, find they must swim and find that the water is infested with sharks.
>
> It is of obvious importance to learn that the waters are shark infested before commencing to swim. It is safe to assume that this initial determination has already been made. If the waters were clearly not shark infested, this would be of little interest or value. If the waters were shark infested, the naive swimmer is by now probably learning how to swim with sharks.
>
> Finally swimming with sharks is like any other skill: it cannot be learned from books alone; the novice must practice in order to develop the skill. The following rules simply set forth the fundamental principles which, if followed, will make it possible to survive while becoming an expert through practice.

© 1973 by the University of Chicago. all rights reserved. Reprinted with permission

Rules

1. *Assume unidentified fish are sharks.* Not all sharks look like sharks, and some fish which are not sharks sometimes act like sharks. Unless you have witnessed docile behavior in the presence of shed blood on more than one occasion, it is best to assume an unknown species is a shark. Inexperienced swimmers have been badly mangled by assuming that docile behavior in the absence of blood indicates that the fish is not a shark.

2. *Do not bleed.* It is a cardinal principle that if you are injured either by accident or by intent you must not bleed. Experience shows that bleeding prompts an even more aggressive attack and will often provoke the participation of sharks which are uninvolved or, as noted above, are usually docile.

Admittedly, it is difficult not to bleed when injured. Indeed, at first this may seem impossible. Diligent practice, however, will permit the experienced swimmer to sustain a serious laceration without bleeding and without even exhibiting any loss of composure. This hemostatic reflex can in part be conditioned, but there may be constitutional aspects as well. Those who cannot learn to control their bleeding should not attempt to swim with sharks, for the peril is too great.

The control of bleeding has a positive protective element for the swimmer. The shark will be confused as to whether or not his attack has injured you, and confusion is to the swimmer's advantage. On the other hand, the shark may know he has injured you and be puzzled as to why you do not bleed or show distress. This also has a profound effect on sharks. They begin questioning their own potency or, alternatively, believe the swimmer to have supernatural powers.

3. *Counter any aggression promptly.* Sharks rarely attack a swimmer without warning. Usually there is some tentative, exploratory aggressive action. It is important that the swimmer recognizes that this behavior is a prelude to an attack and takes prompt and vigorous remedial action. The appropriate counter move is a sharp blow to the nose.

Almost invariably this will prevent a full-scale attack, for it makes it clear that you understand the shark's intentions and are prepared to use whatever force is necessary to repel his aggressive actions.

Some swimmers mistakenly believe that an ingratiating attitude will dispel an attack under these circumstances. This is not correct; such a response provokes a shark attack. Those who hold this erroneous view can usually be identified by their missing limb.

4. *Get out if someone is bleeding.* If a swimmer (or shark) has been injured and is bleeding, get out of the water promptly. The presence of blood and the thrashing of water will elicit aggressive behavior even in the most docile sharks. This latter group, poorly skilled in attacking, often behave irrationally and may attack uninvolved swimmers or sharks. Some are so inept that in the confusion they injure themselves.

No useful purpose is served in attempting to rescue the injured swimmer. He either will or will not survive the attack, and your intervention cannot protect him once blood has been shed. Those who survive such an attack rarely venture to swim with sharks again, an attitude which is readily understandable.

The lack of effective countermeasures to a fully developed shark attack emphasizes the importance of earlier rules.

5. *Use anticipatory retaliation.* A constant danger to the skilled swimmer is that the sharks will forget that the swimmer is skilled and may attack in error. Some sharks have notoriously poor memories in this regard. The skilled swimmer should engage in these activities periodically, and the periods should be less than the memory span of the sharks. Thus, it is not possible to state fixed intervals. The procedure may need to be repeated frequently with forgetful sharks and need be done only once for sharks with total recall.

The procedure is essentially the same as described in rule 3—a sharp blow to the nose. Here, however, the blow is unexpected and serves to remind the shark that you are both alert and unafraid. Swimmers should take care not to injure the shark and draw blood during this exercise for two reasons: First, sharks often bleed profusely, and this leads to the chaotic situation described under rule 4. Second, if swimmers act in this fashion it may not be possible to distinguish swimmers from sharks. Indeed, renegade swimmers are far worse than sharks, for none of the rules or measures described here is effective in controlling their aggressive behavior.

6. *Disorganize an organized attack.* Usually sharks are sufficiently self-centered that they do not act in concert against a swimmer. This lack of organization greatly reduces the risk of swimming among sharks. However, upon occasion the sharks may launch a coordinated attack upon a swimmer or even upon one of their number. While the latter event is of no particular concern to a swimmer, it is essential that one know how to handle an organized shark attack directed against a swimmer.

The proper strategy is diversion. Sharks can be diverted from their organized attack in one of two ways. First, sharks as a group are especially prone to internal dissension. An experienced swimmer can divert an organized attack by introducing something, often something minor or trivial, which sets the sharks to fighting among themselves. Usually, by the time the internal conflict is settled the sharks cannot even recall what they were setting about to do, much less get organized to do it.

A second mechanism of diversion is to introduce something which so enrages the members of the group that they begin to lash out in all directions, even attacking inanimate objects in their fury.

What should be introduced? Unfortunately, different things prompt internal dissension or blind fury in different groups of sharks. Here one must be experienced in dealing with a given group of sharks, for what enrages one group will pass unnoticed by another.

It is scarcely necessary to state that it is unethical for a swimmer under attack by a group of sharks to counter the attack by diverting them to another swimmer. It is, however, common to see this is done by novice swimmers and by sharks when they fall under concerted attack.[3]

There are some very interesting points contained in this essay. Keep them in mind as we look at some specific strategies for functioning in the political arena.

Twelve Key Strategies

As we discuss how to more effectively deal with the organization's political environment and how to cope with the various combinations of the passive-aggressive challenges there are twelve key strategies to help not only weather the challenges, but also move ahead and be successful.

While we cannot guarantee that they will rival the thrill of swimming the sharks, we view them as realistic and unfortunately tested in today's environment. All of these suggestions are based on a positive and proactive approach to maintaining the change leaders well-being in the midst of a highly charged political attack.

The twelve strategies that we will cover in detail are:

+ be patient,
+ maintain your sense of perspective,
+ identify and work with the power people,
+ maintain good communications,
+ avoid isolation,
+ know the "rules of the game,"
+ maintain high energy,
+ be directly involved,
+ manage your ego,
+ maintain a sense of trust,
+ maintain your sense of humor, and
+ use your silver bullets wisely.

Be Patient

When you find yourself in the midst of a political situation, the first important strategy is *patience*. We are not talking about procrastination; that can be deadly. However, rash responses can be deadly too. Analyze the situation. Gather data. Take time to separate the wheat from the chaff. For example, see if you are facing one of the four types of "Yes, but" situations described above.

This is especially important when you are managing dedicated, but organizationally immature people. They will often inject a false sense of urgency into situations. We have seen people at first ignore that they were in a highly political situation, and then, upon finally recognizing it, run around shouting about the situation or crying for help. The key is to be patient and to assess the situation accurately.

Maintain Your Sense of Perspective

Another of those classics of photocopy graffiti is, "When you are up to your tail in alligators, it is hard to remember that your first objective was to drain the swamp." Yet, it is critical that we maintain a sense of perspective about events that occur and problems that arise. One trick we use is to ask ourselves,

> Is this really a life-affecting event? Six months from now, will whatever we do about this really make any difference? In fact, will we even remember this six months from now?

Incidentally, this is a good stress management technique when we find ourselves losing perspective over something minor like having to wait in line. In a similar vein, we often attempt to calm others a bit with something like the following,

> Look, no matter what we decide to do about this, the sun is still going to rise in the east tomorrow and set in the west, and we are going to be here to see them both. The fate of Western civilization does not hang on this decision. Now, let's get on with it.

It may be necessary for the change leader to gain support from others, but you cannot be identified as the little boy who cried wolf once too often. Reserve for the truly strategic times the support of those powerful leaders who can really help you. Do not use up your credibility on minor skirmishes.

Identify and Work with the Power People

All organizations have "power" people. Some have formal titles that convey power, role, and authority. Others are the informal "movers and shakers" who make things happen within the organization. One key strategy for the change leader is to list all the people who are interested in the project or effort, including those in both formal and informal power positions. Once the list is complete, mark the list according to a set of criteria that is suitable to your situation. Include people who (A) will directly use the "product" on a day-to-day basis, (B) are leaders of the people who use the product on a day-to-day

Names	A	B	C	D	E	F	G

Table 9.1. Power assessment worksheet.

basis, (C) have formal organizational power, (D) have informal organizational power, and (E) are highly respected within the institution. Table 9.1 is a worksheet for you to begin to identify the power people within your organization. There are two additional columns included for you to add your own criteria to the power-based people list.

Maintain Good Communications

One can never overemphasize the importance of good communications throughout any type of change process, but it is doubly important in the implementation of information technology. There are several points to consider. The first critical point is to ensure that all of the relevant people, regardless of their organizational position or title, know what the goals are for the effort at hand. It may be necessary to explain the purpose and goals to people in a variety of ways. It is important to repeat the ideas-purpose-concepts message in different ways for different learning styles and levels of information systems knowledge. For some people, it may be important to create scenarios or stories that describe the new system's purpose; for others, it may be important to talk about impact and build models of what is desired. A second critical communication issue is to give the people involved input into the information technology process to express needs and to build ownership and support as political situations arise. After the input stage and before the implementation stage, ensure that the depth and breadth of the project are well understood and known to as many people as possible. We have seen some circumstances where the users' expectations were not managed well, as discussed in Chapter 7.

Avoid Isolation

Do not become so enthused with your idea/project that your ignore the politics of the organization. Murray Dalziel and Stephen Schoonover said, " A basic axiom of any change effort is that the further away the people defining the change are from the people who have to live with the change, then the more likelihood that the change will develop problems."4

Figure 9.2 illustrates that we must maintain *constant two-way communication* with both the end users and the power people throughout the project. Avoiding isolation becomes very important for the political aspects of the organization. When in a political controversy, make sure you maintain a high-profile visible position as the person responsible and comfortable with the project.

Having a good network, linkages, and contacts is essential. Time invested in building these tends to have a high payoff. Reaching for a book or the keyboard is fine if you need an "answer." When you need advice and support, you need to be able to reach for the telephone. One very important tip: always be both polite and kind to the "little people." The generals may determine the strategic directions, but the sergeants run the army!

Avoiding Isolation

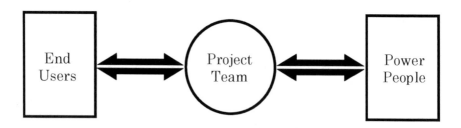

Figure 9.2. Need for constant two-way communication.

Know the "Rules of the Game"

All organizations have basic behavioral characteristics. Roger Harrison[5] developed a topology of organizational cultures. In his topology he has four types of organizations: power, role, task, and personal.

The *power* organization is typified by attempts to dominate its environment. These organizations have high control over subordinates, and they have an aggressive response to threat. They are sometimes very paternalistic and jealous of their territory. In the medical environment this would translate into the creation and maintenance of "baronies." The baronies are not limited to clinical departments, but also could be other departments within the hospital or in other parts of the medical environment.

The *role* organization is rational and orderly. Based on its complexity, there is a preoccupation with legality, legitimacy, and responsibility. Agreements, rules, and detailed procedures are very important in this bureaucratic organization. Stability is very valued and these organizations are slow to change. In an academic medical environment, the parent university typically has a higher tendency to be a role based organization than does the medical center. This corporate culture difference causes major difficulties for the medical environment, which has different needs and different goals.

In the *task* organization, the achievement of the goal is paramount and is the frame of reference against which all else is valued. Authority comes from knowledge or skill and not position or power. In this type of organization rules are broken, bent, or changed to meet goals. These organizations are flexible and quick to change. Task forces are often used to overcome role and power in large organizations. Delegation and participation are prevalent.

The *personal* organization exists to serve the needs of its members that the members cannot meet themselves. Authority in the role or power sense is discouraged. These organizations usually follow consensus decision making, and people are not expected to do things in conflict with their preferences or values. Influence is excerpted through example, helpfulness, and caring. Some small group medical practices fit this model, at least with respect to the professional staff.

While an overall organization may have a predominant characteristic, e.g., a role-based organization, different subunits within the organization may have other characteristics, e.g. task or person. We have used a fifteen-item instrument to measure organizational culture in a number of organizations over the years. Generally, individuals within the organization will view themselves as more task and person oriented and their organization as more power and role oriented. This was true in several situations in which all members of the organization were present, including the most senior decision maker.

When a key person leaves the organization, there will be a power shift and perhaps a change of style. At this point, we are not arguing the pro and cons of any of the four styles of organizational culture; we are suggesting that you be aware of the style that is prevalent within your organization and know how to function effectively within that style. Also, when power shifts occur, it is important to identify whose star is rising and whose star is falling within the organization. If you have linked all your political chips to someone whose star is falling, you will need to find a designated hitter to take his or her place in the on-deck circle.

Maintain High Energy

Major political battles require high mental and physical energy. You may need to put conscious effort into maintaining your physical conditioning as a major project progresses. This is especially true since major project efforts tend to impose heavily upon the leader's time, especially during the periodic "crunch" times.

Be Directly Involved

The key person responsible for implementing a megachange information technology program must be directly involved in the project. The leader can delegate some of the tasks but cannot supervise or direct the project from a distance. In other words, delegation is fine but abdication is not. It is important to be clearly identified with the project, especially by the power brokers within the organization.

We have seen situations in which the key change leaders have delegated too much of the responsibility and authority for key information technology implementation efforts to a person who did not have either the competence or the self-esteem to be the surrogate change leader. In some cases, the people who were responsible for the day-to-day implementation had their own agendas that were not in concert with the change leaders' agendas. In one case, the surrogate change leader did not communicate some of the issues, problems, etc., to the senior change leader. The change leader discovered much later that there were major problems within the project, and correcting them then took an overwhelming effort. When change agents are more directly involved, they can correct problems while they are much more manageable.

Manage Your Ego

Leading a major health informatics implementation can be hard on the ego at times. This is certainly no role for someone with shaky self-esteem. There are several issues to which we should be especially sensitive.

We suggest that you constantly keep a list of all the things that are going right. Heaven only knows, "they" will constantly tell you about all the things that are going wrong. Keep a list on your computer or on a pad in your desk drawer. Every time you see or hear something positive about the project make a note of it. This may seem silly, but it can help you over the inevitable rough periods in any major project.

In complex organizations, changes often need to be "their" ideas. Some of the most successful efforts occur when all those involved think that the solutions being implemented were their ideas. This concept can be difficult for people whose fragile egos demand that they get the credit if the idea was really theirs. It is more important to obtain the desired results and advance the overall project than it is to get credit for isolated pieces of the process.

Another issue is taking something personally when there is not necessarily anything personal about it. This is most likely to happen when there is actually a sequence of conflicts with someone else that we start to personalize. The single best tactic here is to calm down from any individual incident and then ask yourself the following, "If I were in that other person's position, would I be pushing for the same thing that he or she is?" Often, the answer is yes. In our imperfect organizations, there are often built-in frictions and role conflicts that will logically put competent, well-intentioned people in repetitive conflict. Switch the people's roles and they automatically adopt the attitudes and behaviors they were just screaming about. There is nothing personal about it.

Maintain a Sense of Trust

Trust is a broad concept when used in an organizational sense. Are we talking about trusting competence? Honesty? Loyalty? All of the above? Our belief is that a manager who is doing a good job should start with the premise that people can be trusted on all these dimensions. At the same time, common sense tells us that we need to be sensitive to possible failures on their part. Any such failures should then strongly influence the manager's approach to *those same people*. The key is that we must not act distrustful toward trustworthy people. This is extremely irritating and demotivating to those people.

Implementing an information technology system is so complex that high trust is essential. This requires that we select and work with people with whom we have high levels of trust. The level of trust will be important as the project enters a critical stage and political forces and processes become more pronounced.

Maintain Your Sense of Humor

We need to occasionally look at ourselves, ask "What is wrong with this picture?" and laugh. This might sound like a childhood game, but it is a realistic strategy. When we are in a highly charged political situation, we must maintain a sense of humor. This is closely linked to the issue of perspective discussed above. It is critical that we can laugh at ourselves and our foibles, both as an individual and on a team basis. The act of laughing together at appropriate things is a team building act in itself.

On the other hand, the smart leader always stays alert to an excess of "black humor" as a sign of unresolved organizational stresses. When there are too many negative signs and stickers around an office, something is wrong. In a similar vein, when deprecating remarks are constantly made about others, especially the end users—behind their backs, of course—this is a sign of a definite attitude problem, no matter how funny the remarks may be.

Use Your Silver Bullets Wisely

An old management metaphor is that people put in new positions are given six silver bullets, and their challenge is to use them wisely. They should not be wasted on trivial targets nor should they go unused as they will lose their potency over time. This metaphor makes an important point, but it needs to be expanded upon a bit to take some realities into account.

Suppose that the new person is heavily recruited after an expensive nationwide search. There may be more than six initial bullets, and they are probably of large caliber. On the other hand, suppose that the person is a current employee who begs for the position almost desperately. Then those initial bullets are probably more suitable for a BB gun. Obviously, there is a vast difference in these two scenarios.

Although highly regarded accomplishments may lead to another load of ammunition being issued, the management of the initial supply is critical. Some of the bullets might be used in gaining top management support in political skirmishes with peers. Some might be used to obtain concessions or resources that will build credibility among subordinates.

Over the years, we have seen many managers waste their ammunition on targets not worth the fight. In coaching and counseling young managers, we always stress the importance of deciding which battles to fight and which to skip. There are battles than can be won that should never be fought, just as there are battles that cannot be won that *must* be fought.

Conclusion

Organizations are the messy, illogical environments within which we have to perform our health informatics implementations. Our challenge is to first accept this fact and then polish our political tools to get the job done. We do not have the luxury of either ignoring or being incompetent at politics if we are going to occupy a leadership position. We must keep our antennae functioning at all times.

In this section, we have looked at organizational issues. In Section III, we examine in detail the people issues we encounter in implementing our systems.

Questions

1. What was the most difficult political situation in which you have found yourself? How did you handle it? With the benefit of hindsight, how would you have handled it differently?
2. Who are the top five people in your current power structure? Exactly where do you stand with each one of them?
3. Would your political strategies be different for implementing a health informatics systems in a role-oriented organization versus a power-oriented organization? Explain.
4. Why is humor so important in organizational politics? What are some positive and negative examples from your own experiences?

References

1.   Dinsmore, PC. *Human Factors in Project Management*. New York: AMACOM, 1984;214.

2.   Slevin, DP. *Executive Survival Manual: A Program for Managerial Effectiveness*. Pittsburgh: Innodyne, 1985.

3.   Cousteau, V. How to swim with sharks: A primer. *Perspectives in Biology and Medicine* 1987;30,4:486–489.

4.   Dalziel, MM, Schoonover, SC. *Changing Ways: A Practical Tool for Implementing Change within Organizations*. New York: AMACOM, 1988;59.

5.   Harrison, R. Understanding your organization's character. In: *Harvard Business Review On Management*. New York: Harper & Row, 1975.

Section III
People Issues

Introduction

This section presents the people issues involved in implementing
health informatics systems. A 1994 *Fortune* article stated,

> Think of how to empower your workers, instead of dumping
> technology on them. To succeed, technology must come to
> the employees, taking into account their skill levels and
> their needs—not like the early days of computer automa-
> tion, when workers often were expected to learn to use
> whatever equipment management stuck in front of them,
> whether it helped them do their jobs better or not.[1]

Chapter 10 discusses the role of leaders and leadership in the
implementation process, including managerial competence, leadership success characteristics, the special demands of high change
situations, and key implementation skill areas.

Chapter 11 addresses the overcoming of barriers to technology
transfer and enhancing productivity.

Chapter 12 focuses on integrating the health-based professionals
into the information systems implementation processes and on
building effective teams within the health care environment. It
covers professional systems and cultures, system effects on the
professionals, and managing conflict between professionals.

Chapter 13 focuses on managing the inevitable personal stress
that occurs when implementing a health informatics change process.

Reference

1. Special report: Making it all worker-friendly. *Fortune* 1993;
    Autumn:44–53.

10
The Critical Role of Leaders and Leadership

Leadership is a concept that has long excited and baffled the world, but it is a concept that remains as elusive in the twentieth century as it was in the sixteenth century when Machiavelli wrote *The Prince*. Machiavelli saw success and failure for states as stemming directly from the qualities of the leader. Anthony Jay states that today "success and failure for corporations also stem directly from the qualities of their leaders. Management techniques are obviously essential, but what matters is leadership."[1]

This debate about leadership continues today. According to Blair Sheppard, professor of organizational behavior at Duke University, "It's not that being a manager is bad or that being a leader is better. It's that the discussion of leader versus manager is missing the point." The problem, says Sheppard "is that there are an infinite number of things that are wrong—and that this debate just takes us further from the crux. The word 'leader' has been so overused that it no longer has a meaning."[2] This chapter focuses on the role of the leader in a successful health informatics implementation project.

As today's health care leaders try to make their organizations more market conscious, innovative, and productive through the use of technology, they are likely to face resistance from traditional hospital cultures. How well they will counter that resistance and move their organizations forward in times of rapid change will revolve around their understanding of organizational issues and on their leadership behavior.

One study of health care executives revealed that leaders often meet high resistance in traditional hospital/medical cultures and environments.[3] The study concluded that the resistance to change efforts emerge in four cultural dimensions—focus, context, interactions, and time. In times of rapid changes, these areas of resistance will only continue to intensify rapidly.

Focus refers to the tendency for cultures to look either inward or outward. Health care cultures tend to be inward-looking cultures that view events in terms of internal needs. Instead of worrying whether a market exists for a certain new service, these inward-looking cultures worry about how employees would feel about providing that service. The sense of crisis comes when an inward-looking culture is forced to listen to the external environment. Inward-looking cultures actively resist change. Innovative leaders who enter such cultures are viewed as dangerous heretics, outsiders, and threats to the culture's existence.

Contexts provide the background from which events are interpreted. They determine whether the culture will be more relationship oriented or more data oriented. Traditional health care cultures are organized around processes. Their primary concern is to interpret events in terms of "how things are done." Any change that requires altering these habits or customs is resisted. Cultures that are built around processes would rather lose money than change the traditions they have developed over time, since relationships are the backdrop, the constant, against which events are measured and interpreted.

Traditional health care cultures tend to regulate *interactions*. Teamwork is stressed, and people are expected to be part of an organizational family. People do not dare to question the way things are done in traditional cultures because to do so is to question their family's intelligence. Even useless and wasteful procedures may be continued because no one may be willing to question their appropriateness.

In the *time* dimension, health care environments tend to be described as moving at a slow pace in an organizational sense and looking into the past. People in some health care organizations commonly complain, "It takes forever to get a decision around here!"

Today's health care leaders are supposed to lead in cultures with these types of resistance factors. The leadership challenges they face are many and difficult.

Current Medical Informatics Leadership Issues

The converging of more and more sophisticated information technologies with the frustration of finding information in the vast volumes of health data led to a new discipline, *medical informatics*. The term was coined by Dr. Jan H. van Bemmel of Erasmus University in The Netherlands. Not only is the term new, but the concept of integrated information and the effective management of these resources is also relatively new. From the beginning of the growth of information management, the medical informatics area has had a desperate need for leaders.

Who are the leaders of the informatics thrusts in our health care institutions today? The current leaders come from a variety of disciplines that are vying for the informatics leadership role in health-related organizations. The information leaders are computer-based professionals; library-based professionals; technically educated professionals, but not in information; informatics professionals; and, finally, the tinkerers. Each group has a different philosophy. Who the leader is—and where he or she came from— will have an impact on the leadership process.

Computer-Based Professionals

There are many people trained in data processing and information systems. They have occupied job titles such as systems analysts, programmers, designers, system engineers, and system managers. Those in the business for more than ten years often have an experience base of centralized computing. They often possess a heavy bias toward "big iron" solutions to information problems. In the new environment, with the users able to do more and more information processing, the computer-based people argue that they are the most capable of leading organizations of any and all types to achieve their visions. They say they can do this because the flow of the electronic information is more important than the content. They can always work with the content people to pick up the idiosyncrasies of a particular area. They seek to gain control ultimately over anything combining electronics and information, including telephone systems and television systems. Their motto is, "If it's data, we can do it." This is a large group of people that crosses all industries, and their salaries are relatively high. Many in this group suffer from an external perception of low respect relative to other professions.

Library-Based Professionals

Librarians have been trained to manage the content of information and are traditionally known for their user orientation and interactions. They view the information direction as managing the "knowledge" of the universe; therefore, they do not usually focus on the electronic methods of information transfer. Librarians are few in number compared with the computer-based professionals and usually earn less than the computer-trained people. They also suffer from an external perception of lack of power.

Technically Educated/Trained Professionals, but Not in Information

These people are educated in one of the health areas, e.g., as physicians, dentists, nurses, pharmacists, researchers, etc. They have become interested in the information management area and have decided to change the main thrust of their careers. They wish to make the information profession their primary focus and their area of initial expertise the secondary. They have taken some classes, purchased computers to learn by experience, and have generally committed to their new direction. However, they are not professionals in any of the information-based professions, especially in terms of the breadth of their theoretical knowledge. They believe that their content base coupled with their information systems knowledge—which is often not as good as they think it is—makes them ideal leaders for major health informatics program.

There is a subgroup within this category made up of professionally educated people, especially physicians, who are asked to become the champions for a rather complex information system implementation effort. System champions view their primary role in terms of their educational background and their temporary role with the system implementation as a secondary role. They usually assume this secondary role to help facilitate the effective implementation and use of the new information management system. System champions will for the most part always maintain their primary role and will use their expertise from their primary role as a source of power to facilitate better working relationships within the total organization.

Informatics Educated/Trained Professionals

People in this group come from all of the groups named above—computer trained, librarians, physicians, nurses, dentists, pharmacists, researchers, etc. They have an additional master's or doctorate degree in the area of medical informatics. They believe they are the best leaders since they have the blend of content knowledge and information knowledge. They are still few in number, but their ranks are growing yearly. They are pioneers in a new profession.

The Tinkerers

People in this group come from all of the groups named above—computer trained, librarians, physicians, nurses, dentists, pharmacists, researchers, etc. They generally flit from pillar to post and cannot decide what they want to do when they grow up. They are typically unwilling to make the commitments—such as getting training or giving up other activities—necessary to acquire adequate expertise in the health informatics area. If from a content background, they are often a form of "idiot savant" in the information area in the sense of having a very deep knowledge in an extremely narrow area. They often delude themselves and others as to the extent of their knowledge in the information area. If denied a formal leadership role, they can often become potent thorns in the sides of the legitimate leaders as they often know just enough to be dangerous.

Organizational Legitimization of Leaders

Different organizations have different ways of legitimizing and instituting change and supporting the leader. Some organizations prefer that the most senior person in the change effort has M.D. credentials. At other organizations, the person has the title of the chief information officer (CIO). The question comes up over and over, what is the appropriate educational and training background for a CIO.

Often organizational leadership issues are not settled promptly but are allowed to fester. Some of these issues arise because of a conflict between the traditional organizational structures and the type of systems that are needed for the future. Medical libraries and librarians are particularly vulnerable to these issues. In some university settings, the medical library reports to the university librarian rather than to anyone in the health center. However, the attention of the university librarians is usually focused on education and research and not on clinical or patient-directed information services. On the other hand, the computer people argue that more and more library resources are electronic and that they know how to handle the new technologies better than the library staff; therefore, the library should report to them. Left unsettled, these kinds of questions can leave a large leadership vacuum.

To bypass these organizational questions, several organizations have evolved a concept of introducing change into a relatively small unit, which is then responsible for devolving the change to the total organization. In this model, the day-to-day practices of the institution are not initially affected.

Let's look at two organizations that have followed this model. The three senior people in organization A created a vision with the help of an external consulting group. They then hired a person to head the applied informatics program that was responsible for involving the physicians and nurses in the development of a clinical information system. Once the specifications were agreed to, the hospital information systems people then assumed the responsibility for the day-to-day operations. This model has worked successfully because of two major facts: (1) the three senior leaders of the organization created the vision, and (2) they agreed on the person who would directly operationalize that vision. The organizational leaders have supported the change leader through both very positive and negative circumstances.

Organization B started with a very similar model. The vision of the future was created by the end users and the change leader. The total organizational leadership was involved and supportive of the project, but they were never truly committed to the project. When the inevitable difficulties arose, rather than supporting the change leader, the senior leadership started appointing ad hoc committees to look at strategy, directions, etc. Without the strong backing of the senior leadership, the informatics leader lost credibility and the project floundered, disappointing the end users greatly.

The organizations that we have seen as the most successful are those that focus on the win-win aspects of the human-information - technology systems and not on who is in charge of the program or department. The traditional "who is in charge" or reporting relationship approach is a win-lose power struggle model by its very nature. Organizations that are in the middle of this type of win-lose power struggle need first to stop and look at their total organizational vision and second determine what model is going to be the most effective in attaining the vision as rapidly as possible with as little organizational trauma as possible. Once this is determined, they need to move as rapidly as possible to establish the new organizational system and clearly and firmly tell those engaged in win-lose power struggles that a new day is dawning. The message needs to be that the organization needs *all* the people working toward the common vision, not defending fiefdoms, and that the organization is moving on with or without them.

People from any of the backgrounds described above can potentially lead a health informatics change effort if they possess the leadership qualities we will outline in this chapter. However, each of the different groups may bring a slightly different orientation to the implementation process.

Management: Competence and Responsibilities

When we talk about the *management* of organizations, we are typically lumping together at least two quite different major concepts, *administration* and *leadership*. Different management writers have different definitions for these two concepts. Except when presenting the concepts of others, we use these two words to separate two different types of management activities along the lines of the classic Peter Drucker distinction between *efficiency* and *effectiveness*.

Administration

Every organization has a large variety of routine operations that must be performed with *efficiency*—doing things right—which includes the concepts of quality, accuracy, etc., as well as just efficient resource allocation. Processes and policies must be developed, refined, and documented. The resources must be scheduled. The basic goods and services of the organization must be produced and delivered and accounted for. Operational mistakes must be corrected. Taxes must be paid, and governmental reports must be filed. Notice that in all of these examples the time frame is the present or the relatively near future.

Leadership

Leadership is much more related to the concept of *effectiveness*—doing the right thing—rather than efficiency. What should the organization be doing? What business should we be in? The administrator is concerned with doing things well; the leader focuses on what should those "things" be. Put another way, leaders are change agents. The leader envisions a future for the organization, mobilize the necessary resources, and moves the organization toward the vision.

Managerial Competence

Edgar Schein[4] suggests that managerial competence results from the combination of three areas of competence—analytical, interpersonal and emotional.

   Analytical competence is the ability to identify, analyze, and solve problems under conditions of incomplete information and uncertainty. To be successful a manager must take a mass of information, determine the relevant and valid portions, devise a workable problem statement, analyze the data, and arrive at a reasonable solution. This requires sensitivity to the organizational environment, the ability to assess validity of information, conceptual tools for analyzing and framing, and problem-solving skills. This process is very similar to the Riley Associates problem-solving wheel shown in Figure 10.1.

Interpersonal competence is the ability to influence, supervise, lead, manipulate, and control people at all levels toward a more effective achievement of organizational goals. This requires skills in communicating, eliciting motivation, monitoring progress, running meetings, dealing with conflict, and influencing peers and superiors.

Emotional competence is the capacity to be stimulated by emotional and interpersonal crises rather than exhausted or debilitated by them, the capacity to bear high levels of responsibility without becoming paralyzed, and the ability to exercise power without guilt or shame. This requires skills in politicking, wheeling

The Problem–Solving Wheel

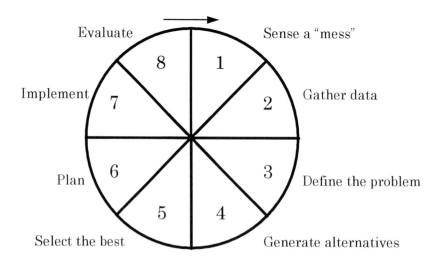

Figure 10.1. Riley Associates eight-step problem-solving wheel.[5]

and dealing, and the simultaneous distancing and involving of one's self. It also requires self-confidence, being realistic about life and self (humble), willingness to take risks and accept blame, and learning how to manage oneself when emotions are running high.

Managerial Responsibilities

In "The Manager's Job: Folklore and Fact," Henry Mintzberg performed a classic analysis of the manager's roles and responsibilities.[6] Mintzberg described three major groups of management behavior roles: (1) interpersonal behavior, (2) information processing behavior, and (3) decisional behavior. Within this three-group taxonomy, Mintzberg identified ten specific roles.

Interpersonal Behavior

Figurehead role. Managers are required to perform certain symbolic duties of a legal or social nature, including signing documents (e.g., contracts, expense authorizations), presiding at certain meetings and ceremonial events (e.g., retirement dinners), participating in other rituals or ceremonies, and receiving official visitors.

Leader role. Managers are responsible for establishing a vision and making their unit function as an integrated whole in the pursuit of its basic purpose.

Liaison role. Managers establish and maintain a web of relationships with persons and groups outside the manager's organizational unit. These relationships are vital as a source of information and favors. Development of such contacts are part of a manager's responsibility in linking the unit to its external environment.

Information Processing Behavior

Monitor role. Activities with this purpose include reading reports and memos, attending meetings and briefings, and conducting observational tours (e.g., MBWA—management by wandering around).[7]

Disseminator role. Some factual information must be passed on to subordinates, either in its original form or after interpretation and editing by the manager.

Spokesman role. Managers are obliged to transmit information and express value statements to persons outside their organizational subunit as well as to subordinates.

Decisional Behavior

Entrepreneur role. Managers act as initiators and designers of controlled change to exploit opportunities for improving the existing situation.

Disturbance handler role. Managers deal with sudden crises that cannot be ignored (i.e., fire fighting) as distinguished from problems that are voluntarily solved to exploit opportunities.

Resource allocator role. Managers exercise their authority to allocate resources such as money, manpower, material, equipment, facilities, and services.

Negotiator role. Managers having the authority to make commitments can facilitate any negotiations requiring a substantial commitment of resources.

Leadership Styles and Stages of Growth

In leadership, there are also styles of behavior. This is different from the competence or the responsibility of leaders. It is concerned more with the observed manner of the leader's actions and behavior. There are a number of different ways to look at styles. We will briefly look at one taxonomy of styles that has been highly researched, another set of styles that has been highly observed, and a proactive and reactive overlay for both the researched or the observed styles. Finally, we will link these styles to the issue of stages of organizational growth.

Researched Model

Most of the research work on the area of leadership styles focuses on some combination of high/low task and high/low interpersonal relationships. One classic work on leadership style was researched and developed by Hersey and Blanchard (the same Blanchard who later coauthored *The One-Minute Manager*). Hersey and Blanchard identified four basic styles of leadership behaviors.[8] The style 1 leader is a very high task oriented person and has low interpersonal interactions. The style 2 leader has both high task and high interpersonal behaviors. The style 3 leader is low on tasks and high on interpersonal relationships. The style 4 leader is low in both tasks and relationships. Hersey and Blanchard say that all of these styles can be both effective and successful for the organization and the leader. The key is to determine the leadership style that best meets the situation at hand.

Observed

Through many years of experience and observation, we have observed many managers and have divided our observations into four major style categories: the on-the-job-retirees (OJRs), the schmoozers, the whip crackers, and the team builders. Although the model presents these as absolutes, there are definitely levels of intensity of these characteristics. Also, managers may well fall into different categories depending upon the particular challenges they are facing. Table 10.1 depicts these four categories.

The *OJRs* are low on task and low on interpersonal relationships. Basically, they abandon the workplace. This is similar to what the Bell System calls, "RIP," for "retired in place." Whatever their staff gives them is acceptable because they have essentially abdicated their roles. In the health informatics world, some of these people have abdicated significant decisions to staff who have been neither empowered or properly trained. The OJRs can be real procrastinators. They often say they are "working on it" and then either produce at the last moment or produce excuses such as illness. Perhaps their most negative aspect is the low quality of work life that they create for their subordinates.

One OJR whom we interviewed was nearing the end of his career. In the same job over fifteen years, he had initially striven with energy and commitment to develop an excellent system. By the time we interviewed him, he was looking far more toward retirement than to improving or changing that system. His biggest concern was not rocking the boat, and he had abdicated the majority of his organizational responsibilities.

The *schmoozers* rank high in interpersonal relations and low in task. Their name is taken from the Yiddish word for one who chats, talks, idly gossips, etc. These leaders often see themselves as team builders; however, they tend to see team building as an end in itself

Task Oriented

		Low	High
People	Low	*OJRs*	*Whip Crackers*
Oriented	High	*Schmoozers*	*Team Builders*

Table 10.1. Categories of managers based upon people and task-orientation.[5]

rather than a road to productivity. They tend to evaluate others on how "people oriented" they are. After hearing a schmoozer praise an obviously incompetent project manager for being very people oriented, it is extremely tempting to reply, "So is my dog, but he can't manage projects either!" The schmoozers can sometimes be valuable in building enthusiasm and support for future systems with their talk of future and excitement. The problem is getting from their groups the work necessary to make the system happen.

The *whip crackers* are usually very task oriented with low interpersonal skills. The image that comes to mind is the rowing galley. The assistant manager beats the drum, while the manager stalks up and down the catwalk with a whip, attempting to encourage higher performance. The whip cracker's motto is, "Damn the torpedoes, full speed ahead." They see the task to be accomplished as the most important part of their responsibility, and they will strive to get it done regardless of the cost.

The *team builders* rank high in both interpersonal skills and task skills. They know—either intuitively or through experience—when they need to be high task or high relations. They empower their staff and they know when to ask difficult questions and when to offer support. They are very proactive in their approach to the future. Arthur Elliott Carlisle[9] tells the story of a manager called MacGregor who holds weekly meetings in which he uses the questioning process to develop his subordinates. Through management processes, MacGregor teaches them to plan, to help others, and to accept responsibility. MacGregor is highly people oriented in the sense of caring about subordinate growth, rather than in the typical schmoozer sense. At the same time, MacGregor is also a highly task-oriented person with a clear view of where his organization is headed and what is needed to keep it on track. Team builders represent mature leaders and employees, who work with each other to make the future happen.

Proactive Versus Reactive

Reactive managers have things happen to them. At the extreme level, reactive managers believe that they control virtually nothing; they are merely creatures of fate. Reactive managers live in the past and the present. In the sports sense, they are very *defense* oriented. Reactive managers definitely tend to be the administrative type of manager.

Proactive managers tend to make things happen. At the extreme level, proactive managers believe that they control everything; they are megalomaniacs who believe that the sun, the moon, and the stars revolve around them as the center of the universe. Proactive managers live in the future. In the sports sense, they are very *offense* oriented. Proactive managers definitely tend to be the leader type of manager.

Table 10.2 has been derived from the work of Oakley and Krug[10] in *Enlightened Leadership* and shows some of the factors that distinguish between reactive and proactive managers.

Stage of Organizational Growth

In Chapter 4, we discussed the stages of organizational growth. It is critical that leadership behavioral styles match the stages of organizational growth. As an example, one health care organization conducted a nation-wide search to find a quality manager for an

Reactive Leader	Proactive Leader
Feels the need to have all his or her own answers.	Has no ego-driven need to have all the answers.
Is telling-oriented.	Is listening-oriented.
Makes all the decisions personally.	Empowers other people to make decisions.
Pushes the organization for results.	Pulls the organization toward a vision.
Analyzes, analyzes, analyzes.	Generates lasting commitment.
Creates sporadic motivation.	Is open-minded.
Is highly opinionated.	Teaches the importance of self-responsibility.
Teaches subordinates to expect direction.	Models self-responsibility.
Is in a self-protect mode.	Knows relaxing control yields results.
Is afraid of losing control.	Focuses on building on strengths.
Focuses on finding and fixing problems.	Teaches how to learn from mistakes.
Is quick to fire those that fail.	

Table 10.2. Reactive and proactive leadership behaviors.[10]

important department. The person chosen had an excellent national reputation and had started two very successful departments of the same kind in other organizations. This organization was thrilled to attract such a prominent person. Unfortunately, within the first year, problems started to arise. Soon the department was in shambles, and the senior leadership of the parent organization was forced to direct tremendous energy and resources to solving this problem. After some analysis, the primary problem became apparent. The new manager had been successful in starting the two departments (stage 1) and moving them to the stage 2 level. This existing department had a long tradition as a stage 3 with very strong barons. The barons made short work of this new manager who was completely inexperienced at the stage 3 level. Ultimately, the organization terminated this leader.

In another example, the senior leader had started the department, which became very successful. The leader's behavioral style was very appropriate for stage 1. As time passed, the department staff matured, and the organization moved to stage 3 of organizational growth; however, the "founding father" seemed unable to grow beyond his stage 1 behaviors. A definite disconnect developed between the manager and his own staff members. Similar situations can occur when organizations move from decentralized (stage 3) to centralized (stage 4) or vice versa. Managers who function well in one environment can find themselves badly out of step in the new environment unless they can adjust their styles.

Tying the Concepts Together

Table 10.3 compares (1) Hersey and Blanchard's four styles, (2) our leadership styles, (3) proactive versus reactive styles, and (4) the stages of organizational growth. This table offers the most successful leadership styles at the five stages of organizational growth. It also compares the various observed and researched leadership behavioral styles.

Hersey and Blanchard[8]	Riley and Lorenzi	Proactive vs. Reactive	Stages of Growth
Style 1 Low relations High task	Whip cracker	More reactive Less proactive	2 4
Style 2 High relations High task	Team builder	Proactive	1 3
Style 3 High relations Low task	Schmoozer	More proactive Less reactive	5
Style 4 Low relations Low task	OJR	Reactive	—

Table 10.3. A comparison of leadership styles.

A Tale of the Sheep and the Wolves

We cannot discuss proactive behavior within organizations without thinking of the metaphor of the sheep and the wolves, which we use in seminars. Over the years, we developed this metaphor to illustrate the differences between reactive (sheep) and proactive (wolves) behaviors within organizations. This is especially critical in health care informatics because people who may be wolves in their technical area often become sheep when placed in management positions, a much lower comfort zone for them.

Assume that John goes to school and prepares himself to go to work. Further, assuming that John has no meaningful prior work experience, he is going to get an entry level *job*. These jobs are characterized by what we call high structure, which is a fancy term meaning you are told exactly what to do. The boss says, "John, I want you to do an A, a C, and an F." These are three small tasks. When John finishes them, guess what? The boss has more A's, C's, and F's for John to do.

Suppose John is a beginning janitor. The tasks are probably offices to clean, floors to mop, etc. What if John is a beginning computer programmer with no previous work experience? John will again be given the most basic of tasks such as making minor updates or programming very small modules. This is often done under the guise of being "a good learning experience." The reality is that often the boss can't get anyone who has been there longer than six months to do that stuff so it goes to the new person. Whether John is a beginning janitor or a beginning programmer, in neither case will the boss tell John to go off and work on some major project for three months and drop back at the end and tell us how he has done. John is given high structure and close supervision.

John has been raised well. He is loyal, brave, clean, reverent, and all those other good things. John wants to *get ahead*. Since Mom and Dad told John that hard work leads to success, he puts his nose to the grindstone and his shoulder to the wheel, firmly convinced that virtue will be rewarded. What happens when hard work is applied to high structure? Success—because you produce results. That is why we structure basic work.

What happens next? The organization is desperate for people who perform well, and John looks like a real winner. Therefore, John is promoted after a while. However, that first promotion involves only a *small structure drop*. No longer does John need to do A–C–F, A–C–F, A–C–F, etc. Now, if John wants to, he can do C–F–A, or F–A–C, or C–A–F. Look at all the new freedom John has! And if John does not like the C's, he can follow the first rule of management—delegate what you don't like to do. John says, "This success is all right!"

The problem is this. If he keeps rising, John will fairly rapidly encounter a *significant structure drop*. Continuing our menu analogy, this means that John will be faced with a host of alternative tasks to do: A, B, C, D, E, F, G, H, I, J, K, L, etc. In fact, the menu often looks infinite. Unfortunately, time and other resources are not infinite. John will have to make choices and set priorities. John may now be the one saying that those below should do A's, C's, and F's. Subordinates may ask, "What about these B's, D's, and E's? Those are all good." John replies, "The world is full of good things, but we only have so many resources. Those other things will have to wait or fall through the cracks."

At this major structure drop, we see the sheep separated from the wolves. The wolf hits this level and says, "Thank God, now I have some room to maneuver, to do the things that are neat and interesting." What the wolf is really talking about are the things that are visible and deemed important by the power structure. The wolf understands the system and relates well to it.

On the other hand, the sheep hits this level and says, "Oh my God, what do I do now?" The first thing the sheep invariably does is ask for a detailed job description. Of course, job descriptions don't tell how to be a winner, they merely tell how to avoid being a loser. The sheep may ask another sheep, "What should I do?" They then pool their collective ignorance and come up with a strategy, typically of how to be a winner five years ago. Finally, the sheep often asks a wolf, "What should I do?" The wolf smiles and says, "I have just the thing for you." The wolf then looks around, finds a number of things that are not visible and not deemed important by the power structure, and says to the sheep, "Why don't you work on these?" The sheep says, "Thank you." and is grateful. Why? The wolf has given the sheep *structure*.

To mix metaphors, the sheep now goes off and works like a dog. All goes well in this little animal kingdom until something happens, namely, a wolf gets rewarded. Then all the sheep gather in a big circle and they start to sing the sheep national anthem. And the chorus to the sheep national anthem is the words, "It's not fair!" When you hear people in an organization utter those words, you can bet your money that you are listening to sheep. They might just as well be saying, "Baaa."

The people in organizations fall into three broad categories, not of equal size by any means. The first and by far the smallest group is what we call the *superwolves*. In a systems sense, the superwolves are mega-changers. They change the rules and even the scoring system. Once a superwolf has been through a system, that system is never the same again. That does not mean that superwolves' changes are all for the better. In fact, superwolves can go down in spectacular flames at times. Put another way, superwolves may well be wrong, it is just that they are rarely uncertain!

More common—but still a definite minority—are the *wolves*. Wolves are also changers; you can't be a wolf without being a changer. But, in the big picture or systems sense, wolves are what we call maximizers. The wolf says to the system, "Let me have a chance to learn the rules of the game, especially, the most important rule of all—how are you keeping score? You let me have a chance to learn, and I am going to pile up the points and win."

Notice what the wolf said, "Let me have a chance to learn." What would the *sheep* say? "Tell me what to do," or, even worse, "Tell me there's even a game." So the sheep are the lamenters, and they sit around and lament, "This whole thing, well you know, it's just not fair! Baaa."5

Leadership Success Characteristics in Health Informatics

Researchers have emphasized over and over that leadership is a blend of traits and skills directed toward a vision or task and involving the ability to motivate people to accomplish the vision or task. Reviews of the literature all tend to demonstrate that no set of traits has been clearly identified as the needed "set of traits" that lead to a person being a successful leader. According to David A. Kenny and Stephen J. Zaccaro,

> One of the oldest topics in psychology is the extent to which leadership is a trait. Researchers have attempted to answer this question in two ways. The most common way has been to attempt to isolate the particular leadership trait. As is well known, this approach has not isolated any leadership

trait. The second approach has been to examine the stability of leadership under different situations. People are rotated across different tasks or groups. Using the social relations model, we estimated the percent variance in leadership due to trait as between 49% and 82%. In conjunction, the rotation design and the social relations model seem to suggest that leadership is much more stable across situations than our introductory texts would indicate.[11]

Although there is a tremendous amount of research and many suggestions on leadership success traits or characteristics, experts do not agree on the definite traits necessary for success. Based on our research, readings, and experience, we prefer to consider success by looking at behavior-knowledge sets. We offer eight behavior-knowledge sets of leadership success in the health informatics area. The behavior-knowledge set forms a behavioral action system that includes task-work-directed behaviors and personal-interpersonal behaviors. The following are our behavior-knowledge sets.

Task-Work Behaviors

1. *Understands the big picture of the new health care and informatics environments and establishes a future vision.* Today many people talk about vision and vision statements. We have looked at many mission statements from health care organizations. In too many cases, the statements are not direction setting or energizing for the organization or its people. The true leaders work within their organizations to create the future vision and they then communicate the vision throughout the organization. The people with this characteristic establish an excitement about the future, and they stay on top of the changes that are occurring. They are comfortable with leading an organization in the midst of an ever-changing and sometimes chaotic health care environment. These leaders know and are able to communicate the impact of information on health care organizations, and they maintain a realistic optimism about the future. They stay visible both internally and externally.

2. *Establishes clear and focused goals.* When leaders empower their people, the people must be empowered to so something. It is the leaders' responsibility to directly or indirectly establish and articulate the goals of the organization. These goals are then communicated successfully to all members of the organization. Remember, people come to work to be successful and to feel

needed. In situations where the goals are not known, subgroups then create their own goals, which may or may not be aligned with the organization's goals. A key leadership behavior-knowledge characteristic is the ability to establish clear and focused goals and then to communicate those goals throughout the total organization.

3. *Has the ability to identify and assess different situations and then use the appropriate leadership style.* All health care organizations are involved with different situations daily. The issues are complex, the people at different levels of readiness, etc. Therefore, a leadership success behavior is the ability to assess the situation and the "followers" and to develop flexible and pragmatic strategies to approach each situation. Sometimes the situation will call for toughness on the part of the leader; other times a more gentle nurturing approach is required. The people in the information systems department may be cutting edge technically, but organizational "babes in the woods," spouting idealistic opinions about how organizations should work.

4. *Has the ability to learn from both successes and failures.* Successful leaders learn from both their successes and their failures. When good leaders are faced with major setbacks, they acknowledge these setbacks and take the blame for failure, when appropriate. They learn from their mistakes and keep going. This attitude is also translated into the total organization. The good organization is asked to assess its performance of progress toward vision and goals, interaction with people, etc., and to learn and move forward.

Personal-Interpersonal Behaviors

5. *Has the ability to develop and empower people.* To succeed in the 1990s and beyond, leaders in the health informatics area must place people and their needs first. This means not just talking about people as their most cherished resource or as very important to the organization, but actually implementing these words through action and involvement. To be successful, leaders work with people in the organization to create an environment that empowers people and prepares them to accept the responsibility of that empowerment. They encourage risk taking and innovation by their staff. Leaders with this characteristic pay close attention to the selection of all employees. They delegate to prepared and capable subordinates. They are concerned with subordinate morale. They encourage subordi-

nates to accomplish challenging personal goals that are congruent with organizational objectives.

6. *Communicates clearly.* When an organization has empowered people—plus an energizing vision and clear goals—then the next most important characteristic of a leader is the ability to communicate the vision and goals in order to gain support of the empowered people. People internally and externally have a high level of comfort with these leaders. Communication is stated over and over again as one of the major success characteristics of good leaders. Lack of it is the source of the majority of problems within organizations. The leader that recognizes the power of communication at the gut level as well as the intellectual level will be successful, regardless of the organizational circumstances.

7. *Has positive self-esteem.* A successful leader has positive self-esteem, which is demonstrated by the leader's behaviors, such as taking risks confidently, having integrity, being trustworthy, being honest, avoiding the need to "do it all" or get all the credit, etc. With positive self-esteem, the leader works selflessly to support people working toward the organizational vision. In addition, these leaders are highly motivated, yet flexible and pragmatic. They have the ability to laugh at themselves. All of these behaviors are directed by their beliefs and values.

8. *Understands and uses power.* Power is an important part of health care organizations today. If a person is to be a leader within this environment, it is important to understand power. The good leader does not avoid power, but uses power to facilitate action and movement toward the vision of the organization. These leaders understand that they do not have the absolute mandate to make changes, but must include all the users as well as the organization's power structure.

These eight behavior-knowledge sets constitute a personal leadership system. This system will enable the leader not only to lead but to lead toward success. Table 10.4 outlines the eight sets and provides an opportunity to rate yourself from low to high on these eight behavior-knowledge sets.

The use of these eight behavior-knowledge sets will allow the leader to have the key leadership skills needed for a successful health informatics implementation.

Behavior-Knowledge Sets	Low				High
1. Understands the big picture in both health care and informatics, and has established a vision to encompass the big picture.	☐	☐	☐	☐	☐
2. Has established clear and focused goals.	☐	☐	☐	☐	☐
3. Has identified and assessed different situations and effectively used the appropriate leadership style(s).	☐	☐	☐	☐	☐
4. Has learned from past successes and failures.	☐	☐	☐	☐	☐
5. Has developed and empowered people.	☐	☐	☐	☐	☐
6. Communicates clearly.	☐	☐	☐	☐	☐
7. Has a positive self-esteem.	☐	☐	☐	☐	☐
8. Understands and uses power.	☐	☐	☐	☐	☐

Table 10.4. Inventory of the eight behavior-knowledge sets.

Conclusion

From the literature, we know that the world has been concerned with leadership for more than 400 years; unfortunately, we still know far less than we would like. In this chapter, we have reviewed some of the current theories and also presented eight behavior-knowledge sets to use as a personal check list for self-improvement. In the next, chapter, we examine one of the challenges that leaders face: preparing people for today's and tomorrow's new technologies.

Questions

1. Of the various disciplines vying for dominance of the health informatics leadership positions, which do you see as probably providing the best leaders? Why?
2. Why are behavior-knowledge sets important in understanding leadership?
3. Why are different leadership styles more effective at different stages of organizational growth?
4. Why is it difficult for some people to be successful at the interpersonal, information, and decisional managerial roles?

References

1. Jay, A. *Management and Machiavelli*. New York: Holt, Rinehart and Winston, 1967.
2. Capowski, G. Anatomy of a leader: Where are the leaders of tomorrow? *Management Review* 1994; March:10–17.
3. Stensrud, RH. Leadership styles for times of change. *Health Progress* 1985; November:30–33,62.
4. Schein, EH. *Career Dynamics: Matching Individual and Organizational Needs*. New York: Addison-Wesley, 1978.
5. Riley, RT. *The Engineer as Manager*. Cincinnati: Riley Associates, 1987.
6. Mintzberg. H. The manager's job: Folklore and fact. *Harvard Business Review* 1975;53 (July-August):49–61.
7. Peters, TJ, Waterman, RH, Jr. *In Search of Excellence: Lessons from America's Best-Run Companies*. New York: Harper & Row, 1982.
8. Hersey, P, Blanchard, KH. *Management of Organizational Behavior: Utilizing Human Resources,* third edition. Englewood Cliffs: Prentice-Hall, 1977.
9. Carlisle, AE. MacGregor. *Organizational Dynamics* 1976;5:50–62.
10. Oakley, E, Krug, D. *Enlightened Leadership: Getting to the Heart of Change*. New York: Simon & Schuster, 1993.
11. Kenny, DA, Zaccaro, SJ. An estimate of variance due to traits in leadership. *Applied Psychology* 1983;68:678–685.

11
Preparing the Staff for New Technologies

Most organizations proclaim that their staff is their most valued resource and then act in completely contrary ways. As health care organizations strive for higher productivity in this very competitive market, it will be the health care systems that most effectively manage their human resources that will truly win the race.

This chapter puts the staff in the center of the circle and addresses many of the issues that surround health care professionals and staff in today's world as we implement our information systems and technology. We start with a look at competitiveness, and move to productivity, technology, and organizational impact.

Today's Competitive Reality

The patterns of health care services have changed dramatically over the last decade. Today, both the number and complexity of ambulatory services have increased. For people admitted to a hospital today, the acuity levels of their illnesses have probably increased, and their lengths of stay have probably decreased. Thus, today's hospitals tend to have sicker patients for a shorter time period. This places a strain on both the employees and the information system. Two of the contributing factors toward this changing care pattern revolve around the issues of cost and competition.

Costs

As discussed in Chapter 3, the cost of health care is a significant portion of the gross national product (GNP) in many industrialized countries in the world, and most are in some stage of reforming their health care systems. While we do not know where health care reform will lead, we do have some ideas of why the costs and competition have escalated in the last several decades.

In the late 1940s hospitals were almost entirely labor intensive, with little capital investment except in bricks, mortar, and beds. Many hospitals had not invested in readily available, and yet fairly old, technologies for their x-ray departments or their clinical laboratories.[1] Today's hospitals—while still labor intensive—are also very capital intensive. They spend large sums of money for new technologies such as ultrasound, nuclear magnetic imaging machines, etc. The technologies used in the day-to-day functioning of the health care environment change at an astounding rate. As an example, we were told on one of our visits that a hospital "needed" one of the new imaging systems and that it would cost approximately $5 million to purchase the equipment and prepare the site. By our rough calculation, the hospital would need to use this system 24 hours a day to be able to charge the patients a reasonable cost. If used much less, the charges would have to be very high to recover costs. Since most hospitals want to have this high technology equipment both for better diagnosis and treatment and for image reasons, there is a technology buying frenzy.

As the technology became more and more complex, there was a corresponding need for health care workers with more highly specialized skills. As the necessary skills increased, so did the need to certify and accredit the professionals involved. Specialization increased—not only among physicians but throughout the total health care system—and so did the dollars needed to support it. Today's health care environment has a higher portion of highly skilled professionals who require higher fiscal support than ever before.

Competition

Before the patterns of health care changed, many hospitals had expanded their physical facilities at high rates. Even though the planners told hospitals that there were more beds available than would be needed, the expansion continued and was, in fact, supported by money from federal and state programs. When the reality of declining bed occupancy hit, hospitals became more and more competitive for patients to fill their beds.

Today, more and more health care organizations are looking to technology, to quality programs, and to their employees to support their competitive positions within the health care system. Many hospitals in major markets are advertising heavily, stressing technology and quality of services as two of the main reasons why patients should select one hospital over another.

Whether leading with the areas of technology or quality, employees are always a key element in an institution's success. An institution needs to nurture its employees in both the quality arena and in the technology arena. One question is how the health care organization handles the introduction of technology. In organizations in which the employees feel empowered and involved, there is a sense of excitement about helping to make the system work. In organizations that do not empower their staffs, new systems and new technologies are not as readily accepted.

People and Productivity

To deal effectively with this competitive reality, it is important that people are involved in any change processes that an organization begins. Today's work force has changing demographics. It is becoming older and more diverse. Some portions are less well trained and educated than others. Thus, it is imperative that health care organizations develop a better trained and more highly valued work force. Organizational leadership needs to directly involve the workers in the change process and train them not only to handle the new technology, but also in basic core values. Peter Drucker has said,

> The single greatest challenge facing managers in the developed countries of the world is to raise the productivity of knowledge and service workers. This challenge, which will dominate the management agenda for the next several decades, will ultimately determine the competitive performance of companies. Even more important, it will determine the very fabric of society and the quality of life in every industrialized nation.[1]

Conditions for Productivity

Jay Hall completed a survey of more than 10,000 American workers regarding their beliefs on productivity.[2] Hall's study had the following underlying premise: "Workers possess both the ability and desire to do what needs to be done, i.e., the necessary talents and motivations for productive effort. They bring the basic human competence to work with them every day and will use it in their work to the extent that organizational conditions permit its expression."

With this as the underlying premise, the organizational environment is critical to high productivity. Hall's research discovered three conditions or characteristics of the work environment that are needed to release the competence and potential of employees. The three conditions are the encouragement of collaboration, commitment, and creativity.

> Conditions in support of *collaboration* ensure the involvement of people in making work-related decisions. Policies and authority relationships that reflect a belief in employee capabilities and respect for their desire to contribute lay the foundation for management and coworkers to join together in a collaborative effort.

> Conditions in support of *commitment* empower people to act on their best judgments at the point of impact—where the work is done. Meaningful work is emphasized, and the relevance of people's efforts to both organizational and personal goals is well established. Teamwork and a sense of community are stressed as cultural norms. The result is widespread commitment to and coordinated effort for the organization.

> Conditions in support of *creativity* free people to look for better ways of doing their work. The task environment is designed to facilitate rather than obstruct productive effort. Norms governing social relationships encourage candor, spontaneity, and even fun in the work place. In addition, creative problem-solving processes, not precedence and conformity with the status quo, are rewarded. The result is a free-flow, free-thinking approach to work and the creative solution of perennial and costly problems.

> *Collaboration* triggers the competence process. *Commitment* supplies the energy. *Creativity* ensures an outlet for people's innovative ingenious talents to be expressed in their performance.[2]

What Workers Need to be More Productive

Everyone wants to feel that they are loved and needed. This is a basic human need. This carries over to the workplace, but here research has shown that workers want a chance to get actively involved with their work. They want to demonstrate their competence to their managers, coworkers, friends, and family. They value being a member of their work group. They want to feel what they do is important and meaningful. Finally, they want to make a difference in general.

Table 11.1 is a list of twenty statements we have compiled about the things that workers feel are very important for success. Think about your organization and rate your organization for each of these statements. The words used—"Almost Always," "Often," "At Times," and "Rarely"—are broad enough for you to give your general interpretation. The goal is not a scientific research project, but a practical look at what employees need for success. You may also want to make a copy of this and answer the list according to the department or division in which new information technologies will be added.

Do you have "Almost Always" checked more than half of the time or do you have "Rarely" checked more than half of the time? If the majority of your responses are in the "At Times" or "Rarely" categories, then these are the issues that you must be most concerned with when implementing new technology. These are the categories around which the technology implementer will need to develop a change process. Some of the employee needs are well beyond the scope of anyone who is implementing or charged with implementing a new information system. For those instances, the senior leader of the organization must be consulted. It is the responsibility of the senior leadership to decide if any of the issues should be confronted directly or incorporated into any other ongoing effort. Researchers are starting to prove that there is a definite gap between what employees are *capable and willing to do* and what management and organizational leadership will *allow them to do*. One study found that if "managers would close the gap—convert the current organizational environment to what workers say they need to do their best work and tap into wasted potential—they could expect a 54 percent increase in productivity over current levels in less than two years' time."[2]

Items Important to the Workers for Success	Almost Always	Often	At Times	Rarely
The organization's policies and procedures clearly demonstrate that people are valued as employees.				
Management recognizes that the organization and its people are equally dependent upon one another.				
There is a philosophical commitment to shared powers of decision making.				
There is a support system for involvement—both logistical and emotional—where the needs of employees to receive and to contribute information are recognized.				
Problems, information, and solutions are shared with employees.				
Employees are encouraged and given opportunities to bring their operational expertise to bear on issues.				
There is a general atmosphere of trust.				
There is tangible evidence that work is valued by management.				
Employees feel they can have influence on issues relevant to their work.				
Employees' managers provide feedback on employee suggestions.				
Employees collaborate as partners.				
Employees feel a sense of community in the workplace.				
Employees have a strong sense of personal impact on the work they do.				

Items Important to the Workers for Success	Almost Always	Often	At Times	Rarely
Employees have reasonable control of their own operating procedures and guidelines.				
Employees have direct influence in the decisions affecting their work.				
Employees are trusted and empowered to cause things to happen.				
Employees are recognized for their contributions.				
Employees feel a sense of shared purpose and commitment among themselves.				
Employees have high energy and purpose within the organization.				
Employees have ready access to the resources necessary to support their job.				

Table 11.1. Inventory of items that workers feel are important to their success.

Technology Issues

The Office of Technology Assessment defines technology in the broadest sense as the practical application of science, whether the results are tools and devices or social instruments exemplified by processes and systems. In health care, technology refers to the drugs, devices, and procedures used in the delivery of health care and the organizational or administrative systems that support its use.[3]

However one looks at this broad definition, we can say that technology and its diffusion in health care only continue to escalate at a fantastic rate. Anyone who drops out for a while from any of the health care disciplines, from physicians to nurses, from pharmacists to librarians, from researchers to computer analysts, etc., knows the immense difficulty of regaining currency in the skills to perform day-to-day responsibilities effectively.

The information technology world continues to follow this exponential increase. Many of the technologies in health care have some type of an information technology-based component. It is the people and their interaction with these information-based technologies that concerns us as we implement new or changing information technology systems. Most people have the need to keep up with the changing technologies. There are in our opinion two key factors that must be considered, and both revolve around employee involvement and empowerment. The first key issue is communicating with people that there are new systems under consideration and that changes will be occurring. The second key issue is involving people in the process by seeking their opinion on their needs from the system.

With active involvement, people can make any mediocre system better that it actually is. On the other hand, if they are not involved, they can make the best system that money can buy seem poor at best. They can even go one step farther. At the International Medical Informatics Association Working Conference on the Organizational Impact of Informatics, Dr. Alan Dowling from Ernst and Young, Inc., reported,

> Wherever I have worked, I have found the basic issues to hinge around people. For example, when I was at MIT in 1980, I did some research into the sabotage of medical computer systems by American health care staff members. What do you think the probability was that a randomly selected acute care hospital suffered deliberate covert staff sabotage of one or more of its information systems that produced measurable damage? The actual result was approximately 45 percent, plus or minus a few percent. As a chief information officer, I had experienced this in my own health care facility. I was responsible for five hospitals and a number of ambulatory facilities, and two of my systems were sabotaged. I didn't even think of the human component in trying to understand what was going wrong. I was stunned.[4]

Even if the rate of sabotage is much less at your institution, it may still be present. Some acts may be as small as intentionally not loading paper in a printer or leaving printer jams uncorrected. Others may be as serious as intentionally planting software errors, such as the classic Trojan Horse, to cause damage. Some of the sabotage may be organizationally rather than technically implemented. Saboteurs can aggressively "bad-mouth" the system, e.g., "Wait until you try it. You'll hate it!" Or they can even spread disinformation such as, "I've heard that those monitors give off dangerous radiation." We call these statements sabotage because they are a definite effort to influence negatively the opinions of others about the system.

Technology is a fact of life, and it is the role of the change agent to help facilitate and bridge the gap that may be present when implementing a new information technology system.

Technology Transfer/Diffusion Concepts

Diffusion is generally defined as the process by which technology is communicated through certain channels over time among members of a social system. Sociologists first studied the diffusion or transfer of new ideas in the 1930s. Over time, there have been many studies of diffusion among various audiences. Four elements are common to the diffusion of concepts: the attributes of the innovation, the communication channels, the time, and the members of the social system.[5] There is a correlation between the acceptance of an innovation and the acceptance of a new information technology system. Let's look at some of the research on how innovations are traditionally adopted and then see how this applies to information systems.

The five most frequently found attributes of an innovation that affect its adoption are: its relative advantage to the person, the compatibility with existing values and experiences of the person, the complexity for the person, the ability to be tested, and the visibility of the results.[6] In essence, the acceptance of an innovative idea is based on the interaction by which one person (source) communicates a new idea to another (receiver.) The relationship between source and receiver influences the "telling" as does the communication channel used.

When a complex information system for clinicians was implemented at the University of Cincinnati, these core diffusion concepts were applied. A nurse with an information systems background was hired to develop both tools and strategies to explain the system effectively to the resident and faculty physicians. For example, two of the products that the nurse developed were handy instructions on laminated pocket-size cards and notebooks that presented instructions in the manner that physicians wished to be instructed.

Several strategies were developed to communicate the innovation to the resident and faculty physicians. One strategy was "open" hours in which the nurse would be available at one of the clinical workstations at hours when the residents and faculty were most likely to have some discretionary time. This proved very useful in reaching those who preferred to receive additional instruction in a more private manner. Another strategy was the design of a "physician versus machine" educational program. Several clinical decision support systems were included in the system. The goal was to have the residents in the Department of Internal Medicine use the decision support systems as support tools. To avoid rebellion, the faculty member in charge of resident education in the Department of Internal Medicine developed the "physician versus machine" educational concept and announced that he would like to test it for a six-week period. Working with the clinical-pathology conferences (CPC) from *The New England Journal of Medicine,* a nurse entered all the signs and symptoms and other related information into a decision support data base. During the clinical conferences, the participants were given the CPC information and were asked to fill out a survey form that collected their diagnoses, etc. At this point, the chief of residency education would introduce a faculty person with the expertise to discuss the case at hand. At the end of the discussion, the nurse would use the computer to display the information that the decision support system had generated regarding the case. Also, drawing upon in-depth knowledge of the complex psychological and sociological makeup of this group, free pizza and soft drinks were provided.

It was predicted that fifteen to twenty people would participate in these experimental voluntary sessions. In fact, the sessions had to be moved to a larger room as an average of eighty people attended each week. The mechanism was so successful that the program was continued on a regular basis, and more and more technology has been introduced or discussed with the residents, students, and faculty on an ongoing basis. In the diffusion of a technology—in this case, decision support systems—philosophies and tactics that are on course with the intended target group not only will help facilitate the acceptance of a new idea or system, but also can be fun.

Although this is one example of the effective diffusion of technology, it follows the research that says repeatedly that a high degree of participation in decisions, clear understanding of the potential benefit of the technology to the person, and active involvement in the process increase the potential for acceptance and decrease the probability for resistance to the process.

Stages of Technology Transfer

The stages of technology transfer as outlined by Rogers[7] include replication, innovation, and transformation. These three stages correlate very closely with Watzlawick's first-order and second-order change levels that were discussed in Chapters 2 and 8.

To Rogers, *replication* means that we use technology to make easier the things that we do today. It is computerizing the easy things and does not significantly change the way we do our daily work. During the *innovation* stage, we begin to see new and different ways that technology could help us. We push the boundaries of how we function within the work environment, but we do not make megachanges. This is the middle level of change that we also described in Chapter 2. The *transformation* stage corresponds to the second order of change. In this stage, we do different things than we have ever done in the past.

One example of transformation that we discovered was the use of technology to produce a discharge summary report. In many hospitals in the United States, the physicians are poor at producing timely patient discharge summaries. The next patient is certainly more exciting than the paperwork on the last one! Yet it is the patient discharge summary that provides the basis for patient follow-up, communication to the referring physician, payment, etc. At this particular hospital, they initially tried dictating equipment located in both the medical records area and physician areas to encourage prompt completion of the task. When this did not help much, they installed a new dictating system that the physicians could access from anywhere, including their homes *(replication)*. When this did not help much either, they started to use the computer to assist in the process *(innovation)*. Finally, they implemented a computerized system to automatically generate a discharge summary from material located in the patient chart, requiring that the physicians merely review the computer-generated summary *(transformation)*.

In implementing a new information technology system, think of the people on the firing line who will have to use the system for their daily work. How will they feel about what is proposed? Does it really improve the quality of patient care, or does it merely complicate the delivery process? Robert Dearden, a British consultant, says,

> Time explains almost everything you do not understand about being alive. First of all, a user sees time in terms of a fairly long lead time. The clinicians who have not been through this before may not realize that the implementa-tion of major new projects takes years. You get them all excited at the level of the 'sell' and then you ask them to wait for three years to see something come out the other end. The clinical users say, "What the hell was that all about? Why did you talk to me about computers?" The second time aspect is that dramatic things happen when the system starts coming on line. Some people will go skipping, whistling, and singing down the corridors saying, "Here is

information that I can actually use for the first time." Now you have a fairly short time window to make the system work well and get return on your investment, i.e., benefits realization. I do not know how long it is, but you will certainly know when it has expired. This is probably shorter than the lead-in time. The third thing about time is that time frames must be what you say they will be. So, if you say from the beginning that it will not be ready until this [an accurate estimate], you will actually look very smart, which is better than explaining why it is taking 50 to 100 percent longer to arrive.[4]

People-Ware

Throughout this chapter, we have presented the role of people in today's environment, productivity, and technology. We can say that the chief implementer is a change agent first and an implementer of the new technology second. Since the senior person responsible for the system is a major change agent, he or she needs to add a "people-ware" track to the project plan in addition to the traditional software, hardware, and financial tracks. For ease of focusing the strategies we have divided the process into three phases: planning and exploration, decision, and implementation. The people-ware strategies suggested in each phase are general and you must adapt them to your own institution and situation.

Planning and Exploration Phase

- Clearly communicate the organization's *vision* and the role that technology and the information system being considered will play in that vision.
- Ask (oral or written) *frequent users* for their feelings about use of the current system and desires for a new system.
- Ask (oral or written) *opinion leaders* for their feelings about use of the current system and desires for a new system.
- Incorporate a *total quality management* approach to the involvement of people within this exploration process.
- Conduct interdisciplinary *focus groups* to gather information from the various disciplines that will use the system. If discipline-specific focus groups are held, then it is the change agent's role to integrate the needs of the various disciplines into the total direction. If interdisciplinary focus groups are held, the

communication allows each group to hear the needs of the other groups; it is the interdisciplinary group process that can integrate their needs into the total system.

- Inform (memos, staff meetings, posters, etc.) in a *timely manner* all people who are located in, organizationally connected to, or are part of the general organization that there is active consideration about the specific project that is being explored.
- Present an overview of the *findings* to key people and departments throughout the institution. Ask for confirmation and clarification of the findings.

Decision Phase

- Include key users and user groups in the process by including them in the *total quality management* approach to decision making.
- Inform (memos, staff meetings, posters, etc.) in a *timely manner* all people who are located in, organizationally connected to, or are part of the general organization about the status of the project.
- Involve key users and opinion leaders in the *decision process.*

Implementation Phase

- As in the decision phase, inform (memos, staff meetings, posters, etc.) in a *timely manner* all people who are located in, organizationally connected to, or are part of the general organization about the status of the project.
- Train people using the "just in time" *training mode.* We know one site that dutifully trained all of their staff; however, the system was not implemented until more than six months after completion of the training.

Conclusion

Many years ago, we saw a cartoon that featured a Viking warrior who was required by his chieftain to write over and over on a chalk board the words, "First pillage, *then* burn!" When implementing a health informatics system, we must write over and over on a chalk board or in our heads that the keys to success are, "Involve and communicate. Communicate and Involve." as shown in Figure 11.1.

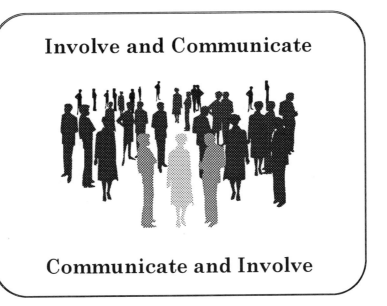

Figure 11.1. The keys to implementation success.

Questions

1. What impact has hospital competition had on the health informatics area?
2. Why is it hard for some organizations to create an atmosphere of trust?
3. Describe some possible types of sabotage of information technology systems.
4. Why is involving and communicating with people so critical in an information technology implementation effort?

References

1. Drucker, PF. The new productivity challenge. *Harvard Business Review* 1991;69 (November-December):69–79.
2. Hall, J. Americans know how to be productive if managers will let them. *Organizational Dynamics* 1994;22 (Winter):33–46.

3.   Office of Technology Assessment. *Strategies for Medical Technology Assessment.* Washington, D.C.:   Government Printing Office, OTA–H–181, September, 1982.

4.   *Draft Proceedings of the International Medical Informatics Association Working Conference on the Organizational Impact of Informatics.* Cincinnati: Riley Associates, 1993.

5.   Gordon, G, Fisher, GL. *The Diffusion of Medical Technology: Policy and Research Planning Perspectives.* Cambridge: Ballinger Publishing, 1975.

6.   Romano, CA. Diffusion of technology innovation. *Advances in Nursing Science* 1990;13 (2):11–21.

7.   Rogers, EM. *Diffusion of Innovations,* third edition. New York: Free Press, 1983.

12
Building Effective Teams of Health Professionals

When we reflect on the changes in health informatics and information systems over the past ten years, we are amazed. Thinking about the next ten years, it is not hard to visualize that we will have "Star Trek" type medicine. In many Star Trek episodes, the physician or nurse has what appears to be some sort of scanner and in a few minutes has a diagnosis, which we assume was rapid, accurate, and physically painless.

We are in a period of fundamental transformations in our lives, both at work and at home, and technology is playing a major role in this transformation process. In the health care area, today's faster and better formatted information is creating changes in traditional roles and behaviors. There have been well defined and traditional roles for physicians, nurses, pharmacists, administrators, and so forth. Easily accessible information can aid in breaking down these traditional roles, which, in turn, causes culture and role changes in the health care area.

Other phenomena are also reinforcing the changes caused by information. Some of these phenomena are competition, health care reform, and legal changes. Health care professionals are trying to determine how to maneuver in this new environment and trying to negotiate their new roles and directions. This chapter is about professional cultures, the impact of information systems on these cultures, and effective strategies for reducing conflict and building teams in today's environment.

Professional Systems and Culture

The culture of an organization has a strong influence upon the systems that are developed in that culture. If it is a major system that is implemented, that system will then in turn have a definite effect upon the organizational culture. "The success of the IAIMS project at Duke has had cultural effects on the institution beyond those of the IAIMS itself."[1] This chapter looks at the cultural issues for three professional groups within health care: physicians, nurses, and pharmacists.

Physicians

> "As the traditional role of the physician as healer has evolved through the centuries of cultural changes and scientific advances, it has come to encompass a variety of functions which both the medicine and non-medical communities alike now associate with the term 'doctor': clinician, diagnostician, therapist, surgeon, counselor, research scientist, and consultant. Of these various functions, studies have shown that physician self-esteem as well as patient confidence are most closely correlated with diagnostic competence."[2]

> "The cumulative result of an intensive program of medical training and a career-long process of clinical experience is that diagnostic skill is generally viewed by physicians as not only their most valued personal and professional characteristic, but as definitive of the healing art itself. Not only would one fail to be a doctor if one lacked the knowledge upon which to make accurate and reliable diagnoses, but it is also generally assumed that most treatment decisions could not be competently made by anyone (or anything) other than a doctor."[3]

Thus, the philosophical background of physicians is that their role is to diagnosis and treat. Based upon that role, they are the natural head of the health care team. Their education process and the subsequent residency training reinforce and support this health care team leadership role belief among physicians. Today, however, physicians are finding themselves more and more under attack from both the inside and the outside. The inside force is that it is impossible for one physician to know all that there is to know about medicine today. As librarians and computer people worried more and more about the effective storage and retrieval of information, it was the physicians who worried about how they were going to understand and consume this information. At a meeting, G. Octo Barnett, M.D., a distinguished professor from Harvard University, commented on this information explosion. Given that there are over 60,000 health-related journals published annually, if a physician read two journal articles every day, by the end of one year that physician would be more than 350 years behind in reading all the information from *that one year alone*. Physicians today are facing a tremendous burden in keeping up-to-date with the changes and developments of medicine.

From the outside, physicians are under attack from the government, businesses, including corporations and insurance companies, and others who covet their perceived roles within the health care system. Many physicians say that medicine is not "fun" any more; that they spend much of their time negotiating about what tests or treatments that patients should have; and that insurance companies are controlling how and when they practice medicine. To physicians, the very words *managed care* represent an attack upon their profession; they have always considered themselves as the managers of their patients' care. Many governments are in the process of supposedly reforming their health care systems, and physicians are worried that the outcomes will be a further diminished role and degree of autonomy for the physician. Many businesses now support the "panel" concept. Under this concept, there are approved hospitals and physicians that the employees of a corporation or members of an association may use. Physicians not on a particular panel may not be available to the employees of that company.

Technology can also challenge the traditional role of the physician. However, progressive physicians see the advantages of those technologies that provide better information and are ready to reshape their role within the new technological environment. Inevitably, one growth area will be the area of computer aided diagnosis. James Mazoue says, "it would be more correct to refer to human-assisted computer diagnosis rather than computer-assisted diagnoses made by human practitioners."[3] The use of the information from the technology will bring the physicians' diagnostic core into the twenty-first century.

Nurses

Most nurses go into nursing to take care of patients in a hands-on sense. The nurses views their role as the real integrator of information about patients, especially for the inpatient hospital areas. Over recent years, the nursing profession has been trying to redefine their professional role. Consequently, the emphasis has shifted from "diploma," hospital-based on-the-job training schools to university degree-granting programs. When trained in the hospital-based programs, the role of nurses was much more subservient to the role of physicians. Under that model, the nurses spent almost all of their time on hospital floors and their follow-up education was on an in-service base. Nurses with university degrees—bachelors, masters, and doctorates—tend to be far more assertive in their health care roles. Today, most hospital nursing departments have nursing research centers. As health care becomes more complicated, nurses spend more time on further education and research.

Some regions have readily accepted the concept of the nurse-practitioner. Under this model, nurses adopt a similar model to the primary care physicians. Nurses have their own patient practice and become the primary care giver for their patients. They refer their patients to physicians only when the nurse determines that there is a need for physician involvement. Nurses formally assuming some of the diagnostic and treatment role of physicians causes a definite role-cultural shift.

As the role of nurses continues to change, role conflicts will continue to develop between physicians and nurses. Any information system that significantly reduces the clerical workload upon nurses will allow the nurse to focus more on management and patient care.

Pharmacists

In many hospitals, the pharmacy departments were among the leaders in applying computer technology in support of their professional efforts. Beyond the preparation of drug orders, the role of the hospital pharmacists has generally been to support the health care team by providing information about potential drug effects and interactions. In this role, they are active members of the health care team. Today, computerized systems offer the potential to both enhance and diminish the pharmacists role depending upon the particular item examined. For example, the same computer system that may provide powerful new tools to the pharmacist may also provide basic drug interaction information to the physician on the floor. Again, the potential exists for role conflicts with the other professions.

System Effects on the Professionals

Computers are found in every aspect of the health industry today. Once limited to the accounting and other business functions, in the last decade they have rapidly moved into the clinical areas. Once health care professionals determined that these new systems could be of practical help, computers became a much more readily accepted support tool. What effects are these computers and information systems having on our health professionals today?

Physicians

Physicians are working professionals, yet they carry extraordinary clerical burdens. A 1988 study found that physicians spent at least a third of their time doing clerical work.[4] Physicians are looking for ways to improve their own effectiveness and to manage their time better. According to Childs,[5] physicians have shown greater support for the integrated patient-centered information systems than many originally expected.

To physicians, the single most appreciated benefit of an integrated patient-centered system is the ability to have timely access to the complete patient chart from the physician's lounge, office, or home. There are many other benefits including nighttime and weekend coverage. Consultations are greatly facilitated as patients are automatically transferred onto a physician's patient roster and the data can be presented in a way that the individual physician is used to seeing it.[6]

Nursing

Nurses are the primary providers of inpatient care. There has been significant frustration from the nursing community for years over systems that added work but did not improve patient care. Recently, well-designed systems have been well received by nursing staffs. As systems become more patient-centered, there is a reduction in nursing report workload and other paperwork aspects of nursing. Because the clerical transfer of information need not be performed at the beginning of each shift, much of the clerical time spent in nursing reporting is eliminated. Generating paperwork can be replaced by working and walking rounds, providing far more patient care in far less time.[7]

Pharmacists

Properly implemented, health informatics systems can increase pharmacists efficiency by creating more time for the pharmacists to work with the other members of the health care team. Usually hospital pharmacies have their own information systems. As these are linked into integrated patient-centered systems, the pharmacists can readily see the patient information that is available to the other members of the health care team.

The Health Care Team

The implementation of a major information technology system in a hospital or other complex health care environment has the potential to build a truly integrated health care team approach to patient care. For many years we have researched the concept of the health care team. Physicians would say that they were the team quarterback. Other health professionals might or might not have agreed that there was actually a real team in operation. An integrated information systems allows all staff members access to information. It is around this information and support of the patient that a true team concept in health care can be created.

Many things can go wrong in physician-nurse relations when information technology systems are implemented in the health care environment. In our opinion it is the role of the health informatics leader to address this issue from the beginning to ensure that the information technology system will build and enhance the health care team rather than cause strife and conflict.

Managing the Conflicts Between Professionals

Conflict will always occur when information systems are implemented. In the health care area, some of these conflicts are covert but are brought to the surface by the implementation. There are the traditional conflicts between doctors and nurses about their respective role on the health care team. There are role changes specified by government regulation and legislation. And there are the role changes brought about by the implementation of technology.

There are six general categories of conflicts that can occur between the various health care professions:

- *Role conflict* occurs between and among health professionals when each group has an expectation of its group's role and other groups either have similar expectation for their own group or different expectations for the initial group. As mentioned above, there has been a traditional conflict between the role of physicians and nurses in health care. Technology could add to this conflict.

- *Issue conflict* generally results from disagreement between people concerning the solution to a particular problem. This type of conflict usually can be traced to disagreements about the facts, the goal to be accomplished, the methods used or system selected, or the staff's personal values.
- *Interaction conflict* occurs when one person sees another person's behavior as being motivated by situational or external causes.
- *Functional conflict* occurs because of task or goal incompatibility and/or boundary role incompatibility. Goal incompatibility occurs when one group's reaching a goal is viewed by other groups as preventing them from achieving their goals. In effect, groups attempt to reach their respective goals at each other's expense, i.e., they believe a win-lose game is being played. Boundary incompatibility occurs when a team member occupies roles in two or more units within the organization. This could lead to real or perceived conflicting demands and loyalties.
- *Hierarchical conflict* arises from interest group struggles over the organizational rewards of status, prestige, power, and money. As resources in any organization become scarcer, intergroup conflict tends to increase.
- *Duplicative conflict* occurs when different units in the organization have similar functional responsibilities. The more that the functional responsibilities overlap, the greater the likelihood that conflict will occur, especially in times of decreasing resources.

Let us look at an example of a professional conflict between nurses and physicians caused by the introduction of a new information technology. This example is adapted from a presentation by Bernard Horak, a health care consultant.[8] In this example, the perceived cultural role of nurses as the integrators of the patient's data/information was challenged when the physicians did direct order entry.

> When using a *manual system* on an inpatient unit, the nurse usually serves as an integrator and reviewer. The physician scribbles something down on a piece of paper which is given to a nurse, unit clerk, or paraprofessional to do something with. A nurse typically "cleans it up" and transmits the information or order to pharmacy, radiology, laboratory, dietary, etc. Occasionally the lab or pharmacy will call the physician back. However, the nurse in general serves as the conduit for the transfer of information. When

nurses fill this role, they learn a lot. Moreover, they have a total view of what is happening with the patient as they filter and organize information from various sources. This is a classic work flow design. What happens when a system is implemented that calls for the physician to enter orders directly into the system?

In one hospital, the nurses did not like this type of new system at all. The nurses believed that the system reduced their role in the overall care process. It took them out of the reviewer, case manager, and integrator roles which they were trained to do and which they had always done. The nurses said their two most important roles are (1) the nurse as integrator and (2) the nurse as reviewer, and this new system usurped both roles.

The nurses were very concerned. In the old system, the physicians were used to issuing vague or approximate orders, relying upon the nurses to "clean them up." For example, the physicians would scribble "d.c." or "d/c" for discontinue. They would order "x-rays" and the nurses would figure out that a T.A. and lateral chest were wanted. If the physicians tried to enter their orders as they traditionally did, they would either get nothing back or something they didn't want. The physicians did not know how to order because they had not actually placed orders before. When the physician scribbled an order, the nurse knew the physician, knew exactly what was wanted, and would make it happen. With the new system, this was not possible.

There was a significant decrease of the role of the nurse as an integrator and reviewer of care. Physicians began to make mistakes that nurses had previously caught such as ordering incorrect drugs or incorrect dosages. There was lower coordination between the nursing plans and the medical care plans. In their new role, nurses tended to show less initiative in making treatment suggestions. In summary, what was lost was the second overview review and analysis by a trained professional. The "second" person had lost the overview perspective. On the other hand, some positive things did occur. Relieved of the paperwork of ordering, nurses had two to three more hours to spend on hands-on patient care.

Effective Team Building

The first question in discussing team building is: What is a team? A team is generally considered to be a group of people who interact with one another, are emotionally aware of one another, see themselves as a team, and work together toward common goals.

Based on this description, one can see in the health care area that professionals function on a number of teams simultaneously. They may simultaneously be members of the nursing team, the health care team, the floor team, and even the hospital bowling team. If the health organization is an academic medical center, the team issues can become even more complex. Are people members of the teaching, patient care, or research teams? What about some of the interdisciplinary areas? For example, in the area of cardiovascular patient care, the departments of Medicine, Family Medicine, Surgery, and Anesthesiology could all be needed to effectively manage patients with some types of cardiovascular disease. How does an information system help the total organization to reduce the barriers to interdisciplinary cooperation?

Before looking at some strategies that the health informatics implementation team needs to address within the health care organization, it is important to look at some of the general characteristics of good teams. This will enable the implementation team to see the importance of dealing with health care professionals in system implementation and the strategies needed to create a temporary team of those people who are interested and who support the information system. The implementers of a health informatics system need to be aware of the multiple number of teams that individuals belong to and develop appropriate ways to blend these people into the total system.

The following are some characteristics of effective teams:

- Good teams tend to be informal, comfortable, and relaxed. There are no obvious tensions. It is a working atmosphere in which people are involved and interested.
- There is a lot of discussion in which virtually everyone participates, but the discussion remains pertinent to the task of the group.
- The task or the object of the group is well understood and accepted by the members.
- Members respect and listen to each other. The discussion does not have the quality of jumping from one idea to another unrelated one. Every idea is given a hearing. People are not

afraid of appearing foolish by putting forth a creative thought even if it seems fairly extreme.

* If there is disagreement, the group is comfortable with this. It shows no signs of having to avoid conflict or to keep everything on a plane of sweetness and light. Disagreements are not suppressed or overridden by premature group action.
* On the other hand, there is no tyranny of the minority. Individuals who disagree do not appear to be trying to dominate the group or to express hostility.
* Criticism is frequent, frank, and relatively comfortable. There is little evidence of personal attack, either openly or in a hidden fashion.
* People are free in expressing their feelings as well as their ideas, both on the problem and on the group process being used.
* When action is taken, clear assignments are made and accepted.

This is a very important list. It not only describes a good team, it also gives substantial insight into building a good team. Attitudes and behaviors that foster the characteristics listed above are positive; attitudes and behaviors that don't are negative.

The Sled Dog Model

Team work does not come about overnight when you bring together people unused to working together. We always think of the initial stages in terms of the four-step sled dog model:

* *Sniffing.* When strange dogs are brought together, the first thing that happens is a lot of mutual sniffing. Among people, we see the same thing happen. Who are you? Who do you know that I know? Humans, having a few resources that sled dogs don't, often do some pre-sniffing when they learn they have been appointed to a team. They start calling around to see who knows what about some of the other people named to the group.
* *Growling.* Depending upon the overall culture and the cultures of the subgroups represented, some growling may occur as some of the members test the toughness of the other members. Often this is an attempt to determine what the pecking order will be within the group. The timid souls may effectively withdraw if the growling is extensive. If someone in the group does not have effective leadership and/or

facilitative skills, the group may stall for a long period at this stage.

- *Acceptance.* Assuming that there are no truly vicious dogs in the group, things typically settle down, and the dogs learn how to function in proximity to one another. They may even start to play together. In the same way, as the people get to know each other, they typically come to accept each other and settle down as a group. Again, facilitation is important at this stage. The smart leader often presents a few small problems that can lead to quick small successes. This can start to build the positive feelings of "team."

- *Pulling together.* Now the dogs learn to pull together and function as a team. The roles of the various dogs are established, and a solid culture emerges. In just the same way, the people learn to self-identify as team members and pull together. The team—dogs or humans—starts to think about winning the race.

Conclusion

For a long time people have referred to the "health care team." In some circumstances these were true teams with all of the supportive interlinks and connections. In other cases, the name was a misnomer. The group was not a team in any true sense of the word, but merely a collection of individuals focused on helping the patient. In this latter group, the usual supportive team links and interconnections are not present.

In tomorrow's health care environment, it will be essential that the health care team become a true team. Information systems can play a major role in providing information and resources to support that future health care team, once the short term-frictions are overcome.

Questions

1. How do computer systems help or hinder physicians in today's health care milieu?
2. What was the best team to which you have ever belonged (in any area of life)? What makes you say that this one was the best? Who was responsible for it being so good? How well did this team handle adversity?

3. What are some of the characteristics of a successful health care team?
4. How will information systems change the health care team?
5. Review the example of physician-nurse role conflict presented in this chapter. Was this a good information systems implementation? What things might have been done to reduce the conflicts described?

References

1. Stead, WW, Bird, WP, Califf, RM, et al. The IAIMS at Duke University Medical Center: Transition from model testing to implementation. *M.D. Computing* 1993;10:225–230.
2. Mechanic, D. *Medical Sociology.* New York: The Free Press, 1968;161–164
3. Mazoue, JG. Diagnosis without doctors. *The Journal of Medicine and Philosophy* 1990;15:559–579.
4. McDonald, CI, and Tierney, WM. Computer-stored medical records: their future role in medical practice. *JAMA* 1988;259:3433.
5. Childs, W. William Beaumont Hospital's new generation system. *U.S. Healthcare* 1989;6(3):20–22.
6. Korpman, RA. Patient care automation: the future is now, part 6: Does reality live up to the promise? *Nursing Economics* 1991;9(3): 175–178.
7. Holmes, B. The impact of clinical information systems on the future of nursing. *Imprint* 1990;37 (February-March):39–40.
8. *Draft Proceedings of the International Medical Informatics Association Working Conference on the Organizational Impact of Informatics.* Cincinnati: Riley Associates, 1993.

13
Managing Personal Stress

For the person leading major change efforts in an organization, the issue of stress rises in two ways. One is the stress on everyone involved in the change. Part of the message of this book is that effective change leadership should keep the organizational stressors at reasonable levels whenever possible. However, a more selfish concern for all of us as we lead those changes is the impact of the related stress upon ourselves. We are in a very high stress producing profession with tremendous demands placed upon us. Often we feel that we are not given the power, authority, and other resources necessary to carry out these demands. The end result is that we can feel that we are under tremendous pressure, which creates stress and can produce untimely burnout.

In Chapter 2, we looked at the basic concept that change *requires* stress to occur. Without stress, the force of inertia will prevail. We also examined the relationship between stress and productivity, making the point that stress is a problem only when it reaches dysfunctional levels. When stress approaches or reaches the dysfunctional level, we can manage it or attempt to cope with it in ways that may be relatively positive, such as engaging in reasonable exercise, outside interests, or relaxation techniques. However, we can also try to cope in rather negative ways such as substance abuse, yelling at the children, overeating, or kicking the cocker spaniel. We suggest that you stop at this point and take a few minutes to fill out Table 13.1, listing the five *positive* stress fighting techniques you use most commonly. In the same way, fill out Table 13.2, listing the five *negative* stress fighting techniques you use most commonly.

A combination of high demands, feelings of low control, and a low level of physical exercise can quickly combine to lead to stress-related diseases. As illustrated in Figure 13.1, the biochemical effects of unmanaged stress can lead to actual illness or other health problems, such as adult-onset allergies. The ideal way to reduce stress is to eliminate the stressor(s). If that happens to be our boss, our project, or some of the people we work with, then our realistic alternative may be to learn to effectively manage the stress. In Table

13.3, list any health effects, behavioral changes, attitudinal changes, etc., you have experienced in the last eighteen months that you feel may be attributable to stress.

Throughout this book, we have emphasized the need to be proactive and take charge; however, there will always be times when we are forced to operate reactively, which can be very stressful. As one change leader said to us, "There are moments of great euphoria and moments of great depression." The key for not only the change leader but for all the others involved—from the information system staff to the end users—is to first recognize their stress and then to manage it as effectively as possible.

My Commonly Used *Positive* Stress Fighters
1.
2.
3.
4.
5.

Table 13.1. My most commonly used positive stress fighting techniques.

My Commonly Used *Negative* Stress Fighters
1.
2.
3.
4.
5.

Table 13.2. My most commonly used negative stress fighting techniques.

Possible Stress Effects During the Last Eighteen Months
1.
2.
3.
4.
5.

Table 13.3. Possible effects of stress that I have experienced.

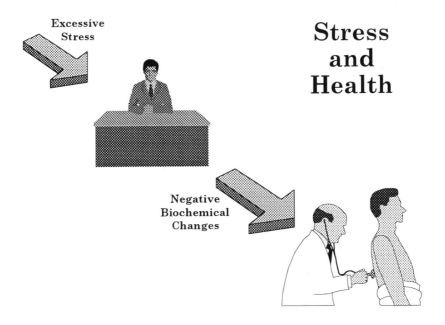

Figure 13.1. The potential negative health effects of unmanaged stress.

The Role of Exercise

The relationship between stress and exercise is an important one, extending beyond the simple concept of just "keeping in shape." Not being physicians, we will give a nonmedical explanation of that relationship.

Most of us lead relatively sedentary lives, doing work that has a fairly low physical component. Yet these bodies—often overweight—that we drag around are not that different from those of our cave-dwelling ancestors. We are physically "designed" for a much more active life, one in which many of the challenges and perils must be met with bursts of physical activity. When our ancestors encountered the saber-toothed tiger, the appropriate responses were what we characterize today as "fight or flight"—either of which requires a burst of extremely high energy. As a survival characteristic, our bodies have evolved over many millennia to support that fight or flight response. Many virtually instantaneous glandular responses (e.g., a release of epinephrine) occur, all aimed at supporting short-run *intense physical activity*.

Now let's look at our professional lives today.

- The boss criticizes our performance or our proposal.
- A peer aggressively attacks our ideas in a meeting.
- A subordinate accuses us of unfairness.

We may perceive any of these examples as the modern-day equivalent of the tiger sticking its nose into the cave. But how are we expected to respond—fight or flight? Certainly not. Most organizational cultures impose a formal or informal requirement that we maintain an external image of calm and poise, sometimes even smiling pleasantly. Meanwhile, our body is crying for physical release. Over time, the impacts of these physiological responses accumulate and begin to alter our biochemistry; then, the health impacts of stress begin to occur. Regular physical exercise can help our bodies to "burn off" the impacts of these negative situations.

Notice, however, the roles of self-esteem and proactive attitudes in this scenario. Suppose we perceive ourselves as great tiger hunters. Now, when we see the saber-tooth's nose poking into the cave, we may become very excited in a positive sense. We may think to ourselves, "Here's dinner!" and attempt to lure the tiger further into the cave, "Here kitty, here kitty." In both cases, there will be violent physical activities and some glandular activity to support them. Still, in the latter case, the lack of fear or panic will alter the responses in a positive direction.

We see this same phenomenon in our own lives. Suppose that we receive three calls a week from headhunters asking if we are interested in a new high-paying job. Suppose that many peers have attacked our ideas publicly over the years and that we have developed the skills to defang these attacks. Suppose that we are very experienced in dealing with problem subordinates. Notice what happens to the stress. The situations may be identical, but the perceptions of threat are entirely different. Linking back to Chapter 10, the sheep cowers, the wolf laughs.

Balancing Individual and Organizational Goals

Organizations are complex places that at times seem to have a "floating" vision and goals. Ad hoc decisions often seem to be the norm. The accepted vision or goal may seem to change overnight depending on the whim of the senior leader. Those responsible for the implementation process may have begun the process with a clear goal and tremendous support from the senior leadership. However, as time goes on and they are doing the best job they can, they learn that what they are now doing is not in alignment with the changed direction of the organization.

When we encounter the above type of situation, we have to stop and do an analysis. If the change in direction is merely an operational type issue, then we probably just swallow our frustration at the wasted resources and move off in the new direction. On the other hand, suppose the change raises some basic value issues such as what quality of work is to be performed. This is a serious problem that we have to handle carefully. If we feel that we are being asked to compromise our basic professional values, we need to confront the issue proactively with those who have the power to alter the situation. If that does not work, it is probably time to dust off the résumé; however, that step should be taken on our terms, not the organization's. For people of integrity, however, remaining longer than absolutely necessary in a system that violates their basic values is an invitation to enormous stress and loss of self-esteem.

It's Only a Game!

Fortunately, many of our frustrations and conflicts in organizations do not involve basic values. Instead, they represent differences in styles, viewpoints, ideas, backgrounds, ambitions, etc. The differences or conflicts that arise over these types of issues are not life or death matters. Losing a battle over which vendor to choose is not the end of the world. At times, it may help to step back and say, "Hey, it's only a game!" This is not a cavalier statement that since it is a game, don't try so hard. Look at how hard athletes compete for victory. The lesson is that even if you lose the World Cup or World Series, life goes on. Tomorrow is another day. Next season we will try again. Play enough games and you are going to lose some. In fact, the only sure way to avoid losing is not to play the game. This is the sense in which we say, "It's only a game!"

Manufacturing Trivial Stresses

Some of us have the subconscious habit of "livening" our daily routines with trivial manufactured stresses. Bob Klekamp, a Xavier University (Ohio) management psychologist, often gives a number of humorous examples of this in his speeches:

- people who eat every day in the company cafeteria and still fumble frantically for money when they reach the cashier—as if finding a cashier there is a surprise;
- people who do the same type of thing in a parking garage, fumbling for their money or electronic card at the exit; and
- people who run around frantically in the morning trying to round up lunch money for their children—who have needed lunch money every day for years!

In each of these cases, the people have manufactured unnecessary stress by failing to take the simplest of steps to prepare for things that were completely predictable. We are not even talking about contingency planning here. Also, note the stress that is caused by these people for others in the system, e.g., the others behind them in line. In fact, some psychologists claim that these behaviors are a form of attention-seeking behavior. If so, a stress price is paid for that attention. In Table 13.4, list some ways in which you manufacture unnecessary stress for yourself—and probably for others indirectly.

Ways in Which I Create Stress for Myself
1.
2.
3.
4.
5.

Table 13.4. Ways in which I manufacture unnecessary stress for myself.

Personality and Stress

Some people seem to thrive on apparently high stress. Meyer Friedman and Ray Rosenman[1] developed a topology of people, classifying them as either type A or type B personalities. The stereotypical type A personalities are workaholic oriented and seem to thrive on stress. You see them daily in your environment. They are the people who press the elevator button over and over again. They look at their watch constantly. They thrive on personally making a thousand and one decisions without thinking of the consequences, only to find often that the rapid decision making has led them to more problems and stress. They give up leisure time and relaxation for work.

The stereotypical type B personality, on the other hand, establishes life priorities and can relax without guilt. The type B person generally has an optimistic outlook on life and seems to have fewer illnesses or family problems. Table 13.5 presents a comparison of the type A and type B personalities.

One of the assumptions of health care professionals is that type A personalities have more health-related problems, especially cardiac type. To help people determine if they are a type A or a type B personality, Dr. Howard Glazer developed a stress-control lifestyle questionnaire, shown in Table 13.6, to help people determine their potential for health-related, and especially cardiac, problems. Each scale in Table 13.6 is composed of a pair of descriptive phrases

Type A	Type B
♦ Workaholic: Oriented toward achievement ♦ Collects stress overloads ♦ Dependent on overwork for "highs" ♦ Perfectionist attitude ♦ Fears not performing well ♦ Impatient when things go wrong ♦ Can't say "No" to work project ♦ Gives up leisure time for work ♦ Hurries in speech, walking, and eating ♦ Poor health habits: eating, drinking, smoking, lack of exercise ♦ Little sense of humor, sees life as serious with difficult situations ♦ Pessimistic	♦ Establishes appropriate priorities: 1) Health, 2) Family, 3) Career ♦ Can relax without guilt ♦ Can work without agitation ♦ Has fun while accomplishing tasks ♦ Less prone to disease and accidents ♦ Has fewer illnesses or family problems ♦ Uses escape retreats for detachment and relaxation ♦ Balances overloads and crises by "refresher" periods ♦ Finds pleasure in simple activities ♦ Good sense of humor, sees life as enjoyable on the whole ♦ Maintains high level of good health habits ♦ Optimistic outlook in general

Table 13.5. A descriptive list of type A and type B personality characteristics.

separated by a series of numbers. Each pair of phrases has been chosen to represent two contrasting behaviors. For each of the phrase pairs, circle the number that you feel represents where your behaviors fall on the scale. To score your answers, add up the circled values for all 20 of the questions. Table 13.7 presents the scale you can use to evaluate your total score.

Behavior	S	C	A	L	E		Behavior
Doesn't mind leaving things temporarily unfinished	1	2	3	4	5	6	7 Must get things finished once started
Calm and unhurried about appointments	1	2	3	4	5	6	7 Never late for appointments
Not competitive	1	2	3	4	5	6	7 Highly competitive
Listens well; lets others finish speaking	1	2	3	4	5	6	7 Anticipates others in conversation, interrupts, finishes sentences for others
Never in a hurry, even when pressured	1	2	3	4	5	6	7 Always in a hurry
Able to wait calmly	1	2	3	4	5	6	7 Uneasy when waiting
Easy going	1	2	3	4	5	6	7 Always going full speed ahead
Takes one thing at a time	1	2	3	4	5	6	7 Tries to do more than one thing at a time, thinks about what to do next
Slow and deliberate in speech	1	2	3	4	5	6	7 Vigorous and forceful in speech (Uses a lot of gestures)
Concerned with satisfying self, not others	1	2	3	4	5	6	7 Wants recognition by others for a job well done
Slow doing things	1	2	3	4	5	6	7 Fast doing things (eating, walking, etc.)
Easy going	1	2	3	4	5	6	7 Hard driving
Expresses feelings openly	1	2	3	4	5	6	7 Holds feelings in
Has a large number of interests	1	2	3	4	5	6	7 Few interests outside of work
Satisfied with job	1	2	3	4	5	6	7 Ambitious, wants quick advancement on job
Never sets own deadlines	1	2	3	4	5	6	7 Often sets own deadlines
Feels limited responsibility	1	2	3	4	5	6	7 Always feels responsible

Behavior	S	C	A	L	E		Behavior
Never judges things in terms of numbers	1	2	3	4	5	6	7	Often judges things in terms of numbers (how many? how much?)
Casual about work	1	2	3	4	5	6	7	Takes work very seriously (works weekends, brings work home)
Not very precise	1	2	3	4	5	6	7	Very precise (careful about detail)

Table 13.6. Self Evaluation: The Glazer-StressControl Life-Style Questionnaire (By permission of Dr. Howard I. Glazer).

Total Score	Type	Description
110–140	A1	You are likely to have a high risk of developing cardiac illness, especially if you are over 40 and smoke.
80–109	A2	You are in the direction of being cardiac prone, but your risk is not as high as the A1. You should pay careful attention to the advice given to all Type A's.
60–79	AB	You are an admixture of A and B patterns. This is a healthier pattern than either A1 or A2, but you should recognize your potential for slipping into A behavior.
30–59	B2	Your behavior is on the less cardiac-prone end of the spectrum. You are generally relaxed and cope adequately with stress.
0–29	B1	You tend to the extreme of non-cardiac traits. Your behavior express few of the reactions associated with cardiac disease.

Table 13.7. Glazer scoring scale (By permission of Dr. Howard I. Glazer).

If you rated yourself in the A1, A2, or AB categories it would be wise to adopt stress reduction and relaxation techniques to assist you through the stressful times while implementing a health informatics information system. The next two sections offer some practical strategies to assist you.

Standard Stress Fighting Weapons

Stephen R. Covey's best selling book, *The Seven Habits of Highly Successful People,*[2] was the result of his research and observations into what differentiates those people who appear more successful in the various arenas of their lives from those who appear less successful. Covey's study focused heavily on the critical role of habits in our daily lives, with *habit* defined as the intersection of *knowledge, skills,* and *desires.* To make something a habit in our lives, we have to have all three. A crude rule of thumb we use is that the firm establishment of a new habit requires twenty-one days, assuming that the subject of the habit is a daily practice rather than an intermittent one. For work-related habits, the twenty-one days equates roughly to one calendar month.

Covey's seven habits are focused more on the issue of *effectiveness* than on *efficiency.* Aggressively pursued over time, these seven habits will begin to alter the ways in which we approach our work, our lives, and our relationships with others. One final caveat: reading a book such as Covey's will do little, if any, good. When you simply read the book, it is still Covey's book, and any impact is at the intellectual level. It is working your way through the book, performing the many exercises, that will make it your book. Learning then occurs at the emotional or gut level. This is the path to success.

Habit 1: Be Proactive

The word *proactive* may not appear in some dictionaries, and some standard computer spell checkers may reject it. Still, the word is common in the management literature today, and we have used it throughout this book. It originated in the social sciences as an antonym to the concept of *reactive* behavior. More than anything else, proaction connotes taking responsibility. It is the concept of making things happen rather than sitting back and having things happen to us. It is an inner-directed as opposed to an other-directed strategy.

Highly proactive people do not blame others, the fates, or their parental conditioning for their behavior. Their behavior is a product of their own conscious choice, based on their strong values, rather than on their fears and anxieties. Covey argues that we are proactive by nature. If we behave reactively, it is because we have, by conscious decision or by default, empowered other things or other people to control us.

This concept is very closely related to the sheep and wolves metaphor we discussed in Chapter 10. Wolves are proactive while sheep are reactive. To use another example, one of our standard pieces of advice for functioning in organizations is, "Always seek forgiveness, never permission!" If you seek permission, the bureaucrats will always refuse it, taking the safest course. For things within reason, just do it. If things go wrong, let them slap your hand. Sheep seek permission. Wolves seek forgiveness.

Habit 2: Begin with the End in Mind

The most basic application of the concept of *begin with the end in mind* is to start each day with a clear image, picture, or paradigm of what we wish to accomplish that day. This is a personal version of what we discussed in Chapters 6 and 7 at the organizational and project level. In teaching time management over the years, we have constantly emphasized that you can only manage time *against criteria*. If we do not have a clear vision of what we wish to accomplish, we will merely find ourselves doing more of what we should not even be doing anyway.

Habit 3: Put First Things First

Habit 1 tells us to take control of and responsibility for our lives. Habit 2 tells us to mentally create a vision of our desired destinations. Habit 3 then gives us some guides on how to carry out the journey more efficiently. Time management is about managing ourselves and the most precious and limited resource we have—our time.

Shelves of books have been written on the subject of time management, and we are bombarded with advertisements for fancy daily planners or organizing software. As Covey stresses, the most important issue in managing our time better is not technique, it is desire. We can read ten books or take five seminars on the subject; however, if we don't have the desire to change, we will simply find countless reasons why each technique will not work in our environment.

Over the years, we have found that even people who set good goals (habit 2), often make one major time management mistake. In setting priorities and then acting upon them, they confound the concepts of *urgency* and *importance*. Let's look at an example. Suppose we start each day—as many people do—with a do-list on which we have prioritized the day's activities as A's, B's, or C's. What

	More Urgent	**Less Urgent**
More Important (A's & B's)	Serious "fires" Required organizational deadlines (e.g., monthly reports) Major project deadlines	Conceptualizing Planning Team and rapport building Fire prevention
Less Important (C's)	Minor fires Minor project deadlines Minor dated requests Some interruptions Some organizational rituals	Trivial requests Busy work Pure socializing

Table 13.8. A time management matrix of urgency vs. importance.

do we work on first, an urgent C or a non-urgent A? Assuming the C does have to be done, the correct answer is one that many people do not like. The urgent C does need to be done first; however, it should receive only a C-level effort. It should be "disposed of " at the minimum acceptable level. We then move to the non-urgent A. Obviously, daily life is more complicated than just two balls in the air, but the principle is the same. Our definitions of A, B, and C should be completely independent of urgency; they should reflect only the impact of the task upon our progress toward our goals.

Table 13.8 shows some possible examples of the intersection of urgency and importance. The key to sound time management is allocating adequate time and energy to the less urgent A's and B's.

Habit 4: Think Win-Win

Many people live as if all their interactions have to be zero-sum games. In a zero-sum game, whatever one wins, the other loses. There is no concept of the possibility of cooperating in an effort to increase the size of the pie for the possible benefit of both. There are actually three potential ways to approach interactions:

- Win-Win, in which the parties involved attempt to find outcomes that will be best for all involved;
- Win-Lose, in which one party attempts to gain at the expense of all the other parties involved;

> ◆ Lose-Lose, in which all the parties attempt to inflict losses upon the others regardless of the cost to themselves.

Many of us are raised with a heavy emphasis on Win-Lose competitive interactions. In sports, one wins while the others lose. We learn to play board games, such as chess, that involve direct conflict. We may compete for limited educational opportunities such as scholarships or seats in medical school.

Win-Win is not a technique, but is a philosophy of human interaction. Win-Win means that we attempt to reach agreements or solutions that are mutually beneficial and satisfying. With a Win-Win solution, all parties feel good about the decision and feel committed to the action plan. Win-Win sees life as a cooperative, not competitive arena. Win-Win is based on the paradigm that there is plenty for everybody, that one person's success is not achieved at the expense or exclusion of the success of others.

Covey's emphasis on Win-Win solutions shows the influence of the work of Roger Fisher and William Ury, authors of *Getting to Yes*.[3] This classic modern work on negotiation advocates "principled" approaches versus "positional" approaches to bargaining. They suggest that the essence of principled negotiation is to separate the person from the problem, to focus on interests and not on positions, to invent options for mutual gain, and to insist on objective criteria—some external standard or principle that both parties can buy into.

Habit 5: Seek First to Understand, Then to be Understood

"Seek first to understand" involves a very deep shift in paradigm. Our normal approach is to try to make sure that all those dummies understand us. We do not listen with the intent to understand; we listen with the intent to reply, which means we are either speaking or preparing to speak. Everything is being filtered through our own paradigms, either reading our beliefs into or blocking out completely their comments.

Covey stresses that empathetic listening takes time, but it takes far less time than repairing the future damages from current misunderstandings. In some cases, those damages just cost money to fix. In other cases, the damages may be to relationships and may be impossible to repair. As we listen deeply to other people, we discover there are significant differences in perception. We also begin to appreciate the impact that these differences can have as we try to work with others.

Habit 6: Synergize

Covey's synergy concept is too complex to discuss here as it requires more far more detail about the previous habits than we have supplied. The essence of it, however, is to combine the previous elements in the pursuit of *creative cooperation*. The synergy aspect is that we are creating new alternatives—something that was not there before.

Habit 7: Sharpen the Saw

Covey's seven habits can be categorized in the following way:

- Habits 1 through 3 are the path from *dependence* to *independence*,
- Habits 4 through 6 are the path from *independence* to *interdependence*, and
- Habit 7 is the conscious effort to "sharpen" our use of habits 1 through 6.

Habit 7 is taking time to sharpen the saw. It surrounds the other habits because it is the habit that makes the continued effectiveness of all the others possible.

The Relationship to Stress

Notice that we have hardly used the word *stress* in our discussion of Covey's work. Yet taken as a whole, his seven habits will have a major effect on stress reduction. Why? As we reduce our dependent behaviors and increase our skills in managing relationships, we are going to significantly increase our *feeling of control*. We do not mean controlling other people; we are referring to our control of ourselves and our destinies. Internalizing these seven habits and integrating them into our daily lives leads to an increase in self-esteem and a reduction in that "puppet on a string" feeling that is a major cause of stress.

Some Additional Techniques

As you reflect not only on your information technology implementation effort but on your total life, keep the following six statements in mind. They reinforce Stephen Covey's work.

- Don't force yourself to be what you aren't.
- Take it easy. Chances are that you will adapt to whatever change is required of you—so try to relax from the start.
- Consider the bright side. If you can convince yourself that the source of stress is useful or necessary, you will handle the strain better.
- Try to avoid surprises. Something predictable is much easier to take. If you can, arrange your schedule to fit around those activities that cause you anxiety.
- Give yourself some choices. Just knowing that you can avoid something that disturbs you makes it less disturbing—even if you do it anyway.
- Think long-term. When you recognize why you are accepting small frustrations (and what you have to gain in the end), it is easier to take them in stride.

Relaxation Response

It is unfortunate that some potentially very useful stress fighting techniques such as yoga have come to be associated in many minds with people in orange robes and shaved heads begging money in airports. Some of these techniques have much to offer us. In *The Relaxation Response*,[4] Benson and Klipper present a variant of several yoga exercises coupled with information as to why their approach works. The process is summarized here as only one way to cope with our very stressful lives. It is by no means the only way. The key is finding something that works for you and then making that a part of your life's habits.

The case for the use of the relaxation response by healthy, but harassed individuals is straightforward. It can act as a built-in method of counteracting the stresses of everyday living that bring forth the fight or flight response. This relaxation response technique is used in the treatment and perhaps the prevention of diseases such as hypertension.

The relaxation response has four basic components necessary to bring forth the response:

- A *quiet environment* with as few distractions as possible.
- A *mental device* to shift the mind from logical, externally oriented thought. There should be constant stimulus: a sound, word, or phrase repeated silently or aloud; or fixed gazing at an object. Since one of the major difficulties in the elicitation of the relaxation response is "mind wandering" the

repetition of the word or phrase is a way to help break the train of distracting thoughts. Attention to the normal rhythm of breathing is also useful and enhances the repetition of the sound or the word.

♦ A *passive attitude*: When distracting thoughts occur, they are to be disregarded and attention redirected to the repetition or gazing.

♦ A *comfortable position*.

The following is the relaxation response technique as used at the Beth Israel Hospital of Boston.

1. Sit quietly in a comfortable position
2. Close your eyes.
3. Deeply relax all your muscles, beginning at your feet and progressing up to your face. Keep them relaxed.
4. Breathe through your nose. Become aware of your breathing. As you breathe out, say the word "one" silently to yourself. For example, breathe IN . . . OUT, "ONE"; IN . . .OUT, "ONE"; etc. Breathe easily and naturally.
5. Continue for 10 to 20 minutes. You may open your eyes to check the time, but do not use an alarm. When you finish, sit quietly for several minutes, at first with your eyes closed and later with your eyes opened. Do not stand up for a few minutes.
6. Do not worry about whether your are successful in achieving a deep level of relaxation. Maintain a passive attitude and permit relaxation to occur at its own pace. When distracting thoughts occur, try to ignore them by not dwelling upon them and return to repeating "ONE." With practice, the response should come with little effort. Practice the technique once or twice daily, but not within two hours after any meal, since the digestive processes seem to interfere with the elicitation of the relaxation response.

Conclusion

Implementing a new health informatics system is stressful. Some of that stress comes from positive circumstances and some from negative circumstances. It is important for those involved in this process to both manage their own stress and to be aware that some of the behaviors that they may encounter are based on the stress of others. This chapter was developed primarily to assist the change leader with managing his or her stress. However, a by-product is to assist the change leader with understanding the stress of others and supporting them in their stress-fighting efforts.

Stress is ever present in our daily lives. As the world seems to get more and more complicated, our stresses seem to increase also. As our organizations reengineer and restructure, we are observing more and more "burned-out bosses."[5] Following the habits of highly successful people and stress reduction techniques is one way to keep our eyes on the ultimate objectives—and attain them without killing ourselves.

Questions

1. Why do Win-Win strategies produce less stress when implementing health informatics systems?
2. How will fully implemented health informatics systems help reduce stress?
3. How does the relaxation response help reduce stress?
4. Looking at your answers in Tables 13.1 through 13.4, what specific positive steps can you take to improve those answers?

References

1. Friedman, M, Rosenman, R. *Type A Behavior and Your Heart.* New York: Alfred A. Knopf, 1974.
2. Covey, SR. *The Seven Habits of Highly Effective People: Powerful Lessons in Personal Change.* New York: Simon & Schuster, 1989.
3. Fisher, R, Ury, W. *Getting to Yes: Negotiating Agreement Without Giving In.* Boston: Houghton Mifflin, 1981.
4. Benson, H, Klipper, MZ. *The Relaxation Response.* New York: William Morrow, 1976.
5. Smith, L. Burned-out bosses. *Fortune* July 25, 1994; 44–52.

Section IV
Managing the Project End Stages

Introduction

As we come toward the end of the systems development process, the specter of "cutover" looms ahead—that moment of truth when the switch is thrown on the new system. Will we experience the "thrill of victory" or suffer from the "agony of defeat?" In this section, we deal with a critical question: When is the project really over? Is it ever over, for that matter? To use an analogy, suppose you had asked ten years ago, "When is a negotiation over?" Most people would have told you, "When the contract is signed, of course." Today, many people realize that the negotiation is actually over when the agreement has been completely implemented. In the same way, we are learning that we cannot successfully drop ship new systems into an organization.

By the time the cutover stage is reached, the technical capabilities of the system are essentially determined. However, the way in which the end stage activities are carried out can have a large effect on how the system is both received and perceived by the end-users. While it is tempting to charge off seeking the next informatics mountain to scale, there are several end stage strategies that we need to follow. The three chapters in this section focus on these strategies.

Chapter 14 focuses on some pre- and post-cutover people issues, including identifying system shortcomings, changes in the work place, continuing to remove barriers, training, celebration of the new system, and "mending fences." These issues involve both staff and patients and, if not dealt with effectively, can lead to major organizational issues.

Chapter 15 reviews the area of evaluation. Does the system product meet the original expectations of the system designers and the system users? What was learned during this process?

Chapter 16 focuses on the new or "altered" organization and strategies for effectively managing in the altered organization.

14
Dealing with End Stage People Issues

One of the central themes of this book has been that time and energy put in upstream in the right places will have high payoffs downstream. Most end stage issues are quite reasonable to deal with when the informatics implementation process has been managed well from the beginning. On the other hand, one of the worst jobs in health informatics is to inherit a project which is well along in the process and which has been mismanaged from the beginning. Here, facing the end stage issues can be truly grim.

These end stage implementation issues form a special topic because some definite changes occur at implementation or "cutover" to the new system. Sometimes the leaders of health informatics implementation projects assume that everyone in the organization has lived and breathed the implementation effort as much as they have. Even when the leaders of the informatics change efforts have done a spectacular job with communication and involvement, the ultimate end-users still tend to understand the informatics project at the *intellectual* level, not at the *emotional* or gut level. Put another way, until the system becomes operational, the end-users are merely *involved* in the process while the informatics leaders are *committed*. At cutover time, the end-users suddenly have to work with this new system and integrate the required behavioral changes into their daily work lives. For these people, the actual implementation has transformed the plans and ideas that they read about from a Level One change into a Level Two change.

On the other hand, the leaders of the informatics change effort are probably so tired of both the large and the small issues connected with this effort that they are becoming worn down and tired of dealing with it. They might also be the type of people who get their thrills from analyzing and solving problems; therefore, they now want to go and find the next challenge and not have to perform a lot of "hand-holding" for the end-users. However, the quality of perform-ance at the end stages of one project can have tremendous impact on the *ease of implementing future projects*. As we move to new projects, the last thing we need is horror stories circulating in the halls about the last project.

Figure 14.1 illustrates the unfortunate end stage pattern that many informatics project leaders have used in the past. Notice that the time and energy dedicated to the project is actually sliding a bit as the project staff is growing weary of it. However, as cutover time nears, "Crunch Time" begins in a desperate effort to meet deadlines. This tremendous adrenaline surge is then followed by a tremendous letdown once the switch is thrown. As rapidly as possible, the project staff engages in a rapid "Flight" away from the system and the end-users. The entire project staff is sick of the system and wants nothing to do with it any more. The only thing that brings them back to it is a major "Crisis" which they deal with grudgingly and again flee. Figure 14.1 shows only one such crisis, but in practice several can occur.

As we have discussed earlier, part of the basic problem is the whole value set under which the project has been conducted. If project success has been defined in technical terms, then a system that the technicians can make work is a success. If project success has been defined in terms of end-user satisfaction, then the problems with the traditional model are obvious.

Figure 14.2 shows a more end-user oriented model. With good project management, the level of time and energy in the latter project stages is kept more constant. There is still a "Crunch Time;" after all, these are human beings involved! However, the magnitude

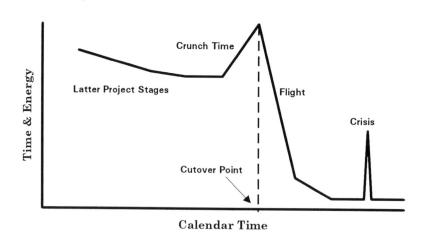

Figure 14.1. Traditional end stage pattern.

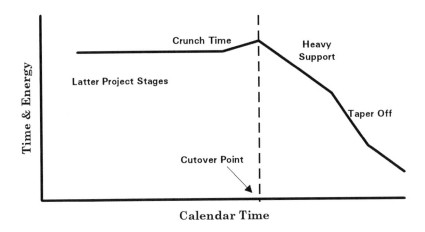

Figure 14.2. A more desirable end stage pattern.

is nowhere near so pronounced. The major difference is in the intensive post-cutover effort put into supporting the end-users as they adjust to the new system. The "Taper Off" stage occurs only after this adjustment has occurred. Even then, there is a solid level of ongoing support for the system. Figures 14.1 and 14.2 represent major philosophical differences in the approach to implementing systems. More and more, informatics professionals are coming to realize that the latter approach is the only one that works.

The goal of this chapter is to keep the people issues in the minds of the change leaders so that they follow the gradual and more successful road to bringing the majority of staff into full partnership with the system.

Training and Support

The quality of the training and support which accompany a new system will have a great impact on the success of that system. Yet, training is often handled as something of an afterthought. Once again, the higher the quality at each step of the training and support process, the lower the demands on successive steps. Good training will not eliminate the need for ongoing support, but it will certainly reduce that need.

Training

While communication about the new system should begin as soon as possible, the actual training to use the new system should be delayed as long as possible. We are talking about the training being delayed, not the planning of the training, of course. The "just-in-time" concept should be applied to the training. The training should occur as close as possible to the time when the staff will need to use the system on a regular basis. One health care organization had a large staff, but limited classroom space and trainers; therefore, they compulsively started training every staff member on how to use the new system. Unfortunately, some people were trained as much as six months before the system was installed. When the cutover occurred, most of the "trained" staff members were completely unprepared to use the new system. The new system had to be shut down and the staff trained again.

We learned long ago that there are two components in most forms of training: (1) technical content and (2) attitudes. Any training needs to be a combination of educating people in how to use the system *plus* building their enthusiasm for doing so. There definitely needs to be a "pep rally" element to the training. This has many implications for the curriculum content and the choice of trainers. For a truly important systems implementation, many organizations may well be better off hiring professionals to do or assist in developing this training.

Another key training issue is recognizing the possible need to do staged training for complex systems. Initial training may be necessary to allow the people to perform basic activities on the system. Additional training can then follow as soon as the people have used the system enough to be ready for additional training. For complex systems, trying to do all the training at one time almost guarantees that most of the trainees will mentally drop out at some point in the process.

In training physicians, special problems often arise. In many environments, it is very unlikely that they will commit to group training sessions of any length. In addition, they may be the most impatient and critical of the quality of any training. The training for this powerful group will require the most careful planning, development, and staffing. Also, it is critical to get the strong support of the informal physician leadership in support of participation in the training.

The traditional training process is to bring twenty or more people together and instruct them. However, traditional classroom instruction is often not the best method in systems which have characteristics such as shift work and moderate to high employee turnover. Classroom type training is often relatively ineffective in dealing with the challenge of continual new hires. Today, techniques such as interactive video disc are becoming increasingly affordable and can provide on-demand training as needed.

Materials

At least some of the training materials should be concise reference cards which can act as security blankets for the end-users as they face the challenge of the new system. Ideally, today's systems have on-line help functions which utilize a hypertext type approach for maximum usefulness. Still, something physical such as a card can be a comfort until the end-user is comfortable with the on-line support provided.

Support

Support falls into two categories: initial and ongoing. As indicated in Figure 14.2, intensive initial support is needed during the period immediately following the cutover to the new system. There are two aspects to this support. One is the overt task-oriented aspect of providing rapid, competent help to those struggling with the new system. The other more subtle aspect is the conveying of an image of caring and support. The duration of this intensive support period will depend upon the complexity of the system, the size of the group, and the level of information systems sophistication within the group.

As the need for intense support diminishes, ongoing support can typically be transferred to a "help-desk" type function available to take calls and talk someone through a particular problem. If the help-desk is targeted to one specific implementation, then it will probably be a short lived desk and its functions can be folded into a more general help function at a later date.

Today, overall support is a blend of initial training, the built-in capabilities of the system itself, the written documentation, and the personal support provided by experts. While there is a tendency to minimize the demand for the personal type support for the sake of efficiency, always remember that there are times when the need will be felt for human interaction about particular problems. This is another example of what John Naisbitt's calls High Tech-High Touch.[1]

Communication

Whether talking about leadership or staff involvement, communication is the cornerstone of success when implementing a health informatics information system. The process is complex, the system is complex, and the potential stresses on the staff are also complex. Extensive and frequent information about the effort under way is one effective method available to address all of the personal security and insecurity issues that arise from the staff. We must be careful not to let the level of communication fall off during the end stages of the project. Here are several suggested types of communications:

- A very effective communication tool is to express written thanks and appreciation to those who have supported the implementation effort. One of the most negative traps that people in an organization can fall into is what we call, "That's what they are paid for." In other words, the only time we need to communicate is to complain because the other person is paid to do good things. This violates every rule of good psychology. A note of thanks which communicates our sincere appreciation is a sound motivational strategy. However, a word of caution in this age of word processing. We must not be so compulsive and task oriented that we send the same quick two-line note of thanks to everyone regardless of the size of the contribution. We used the phrase, *sincere appreciation*, above. Sincerity requires that we take a few moments to personalize our thanks. Sending the same note to both major and minor contributors will be more of a demotivator for a major contributor than a motivator.

- End-users must continue to receive regular information about the system, even after their training. The information could be in the form of newsletters, memos, posters, etc. The information could be on issues that have arisen, anecdotes, feelings, feedback, etc. The content is important, but even more important is the regular information about the system.

- We have talked about staff throughout this book. Now, it is time to "put the patient in the driver's seat" and talk about the patients and guests within the health care institution. Today patients and their families are more involved in their treatment than ever before. It is very important to tell the patients and their guests about the new systems and its capabilities. Communications to patients could take the form of newsletters, letters, posters, examples of printouts, etc. If appropriate, the patients or their guests might be given access to a mock database so that can appreciate the modern capabilities available to their health care providers. We often fail to appreciate that our client groups have ever increasing expectations about the quality of the information systems which serve them. Many of our patients, visitors, and guests are accustomed to seeing sophisticated systems at work in airlines, banks, fast food restaurants, and in the companies in which they work. It is wise to ensure that they realize their health care providers have sophisticated systems at work.

Celebration

Organizations need to take time to celebrate changes and milestones. All too often, staff members meet primarily at farewell parties for those leaving the organization and not at celebrations of organizational successes. We are aware, of course, that some of these departures may well merit jubilant celebrations. However, the successful installation of a new health informatics system should also be a cause for celebration.

Throughout an implementation effort there are many people who have contributed directly or indirectly to the process. Some people are "organizational heroes" for their efforts in the implementation process, and they should be acknowledged and honored. Many people are concerned about the changes that have taken place and need to be reassured that the organization backs the changes totally. Celebrations provide opportunities for those that worked on the implementation and those that are the outcome recipients to come together to laugh a little and celebrate the success. This type of celebration builds an organization's proactive, team building corporate culture.

There are two important points to remember about these celebrations:

- Top management needs to express its support both through its presence and its financial support of the celebration. This does not have to be a black tie dinner. Pizza and soft drinks may be fine. The attention is more important than the menu.
- It is important to stress that this is a celebration of reaching a *significant milestone on a long journey*, not an arrival at the destination. Again, this is a stressing of the proactive, forward looking aspect of the culture.

Changes in the Work Force

The work force is never stable. People join and leave organizations on a regular basis. Especially in larger hospitals, with their high numbers of staff working on a round-the-clock, seven-day-a-week basis, there are frequent personnel changes. The new (post-cutover) people will not know about the old systems. They will join the hospital, begin using the new system, and either like it or not, based primarily on the quality of the system, not on a comparison to the old "how it used to be" system.

If pockets of resistance to the new system remain, they can lead to some we-versus-they situations. Some people may glorify the good old days in their minds and bond together in trying to keep the old times going. In one health care organization, some of the staff liked the computer system that had been replaced more than ten years earlier. Although the senior leader kept the organization moving forward, there were still some people who would gather to talk about the good old days. Although we did not investigate this situation in depth, we strongly suspect that the old system had merely become a symbol for a time when this sub-group felt a higher level of comfort. If these same people were in fact forced to use that old system, we suspect they would have found it completely unsatisfactory—but would never admit it.

Another major change happening in the work force is in the role of the middle manager, and this role is the focal point for much dissatisfaction in today's organizations. The phenomenon of large numbers of middle managers is a twentieth century development, in fact, primarily since WW II. Health care organizations are notorious for having high numbers of middle managers. As organizations grew large numbers of middle managers were seen as necessary to disseminate communications downward and to filter the flow of upward information. Further, these managers were necessary to make all the decisions which those lower in the organization were deemed incapable of making. The jobs that evolved were often thankless ones. Middle managers felt they were both damned from above and damned from below. On the positive side—from the middle managers' viewpoint—there were a lot of these jobs and they paid well.

Today's information systems and today's organizational systems working together have had tremendous impact on both the demand for middle managers and the nature of the jobs. Good information systems can assume a lot of the information dissemination and filtration roles. New organizational systems stress the empowerment of people and the movement of decision making to lower and lower levels. The role of middle managers is constantly shifting from a more vertically oriented role to a more horizontally oriented one. Today's middle manager has to focus more on facilitating roles as the traditional director and controller roles diminish. Those designing and implementing information systems have to be sensitive that middle managers can become very stressed in the project end stages as they suddenly come face to face with some of the managerial impacts of the new system.

As an example, if we look at academic medical centers today, department chairmen are often finding themselves under heavy pressure. The faculty members often feel they are not receiving the information they need from the chair. Consequently, they frequently challenge the role of the chair. On the other hand, the world of health care is becoming more and more interdisciplinary, and the senior medical center leadership wants to move in interdisciplinary directions. The academic departmental chairs believe it is their responsibility to "run their departments," while the senior medical center leaders believe it is their responsibility to "run" the interdisciplinary programs. This causes significant organizational turmoil and pressure for the department heads. New technologies call for new directions and new roles which aggravate organizational stresses.

Continuing to Break Down Barriers

Technology continues to break down the barriers within organizations. We strongly recommend that health informatics leaders acknowledge as soon as possible the barriers that are being broken and work with the organizational development people within their organizations to develop the needed strategies to replace the old ways as smoothly as possible. When barriers break down, new relationships have to be developed. this will require new attitudes, new habits, and very possibly new skills. These are complex issues which are often best dealt with by professionals skilled in the organizational development area. Remember always that when a new system surfaces problems that may have nothing to do with the system, the system will still often be blamed. The smart informatics leader attempts to get the problem resolved regardless of whether the new system actually caused it.

Coping with System "Shortcomings"

Plan as thoroughly and as compulsively as we can, and there will still be system shortcomings and system glitches that were not anticipated. Throughout the initial tests and pilot runs, all aspects of the new system work well; but when cutover time arrives, unanticipated problems arise. Murphy's Laws triumph again! There are two types of possible problems: those that can be reasonably fixed and those that can't.

The Fixable Problems

Part of an intelligent end stage strategy is to have a system in place to capture feedback and rapidly identify any real flaws in the system. The intensive initial support discussed earlier in this chapter should handle the complaints which are real to the end-users but which are not actually system flaws. Feedback on actual flaws should be given to the end-users as rapidly as possible including interim work-arounds or patches and a definite timetable for the permanent solution. Prompt action can minimize the circulation of those rumors of disaster. How the implementation team handles these problems—in a proactive or reactive manner—will have a major impact upon the image of the informatics team.

The Unfixable Problems

The real moment of truth arises when a problem is uncovered which can not be reasonably solved within the context of the new system. For example, the data structure underlying the system will not support a particular analysis, and there is no reasonable way that this structure can be modified. Usually, this is prime finger pointing time. A "blame alert" is sounded, and everyone assumes their strongest defensive positions. This is a natural result for projects that were not actually team efforts.

Suppose we had a truly representative development team, informatics specialists, end users, other key stakeholders, etc. Now it is "our" problem that the system won't perform in certain necessary ways. In some way, "we" failed to meet this need. Without this team approach, it is inevitable that it will be "your" fault.

It is critical that the shortcoming be openly acknowledged rather than covered up. We have all heard the jokes about software companies labeling bugs as "undocumented features." If we intend to command respect, we must both seek credit for our successes and take responsibility for our shortcomings. If this problem cannot be fixed until the next major upgrade, then we must openly say so and provide the best interim solution we can. There is no alternative if we wish to build our credibility over time.

Mending Fences

Even if the change leader went to the Miss Manners School of Politeness and Good Behavior, there will be hurt feelings and peoples' toes will be stepped upon, especially in the turmoil of cutover. Just as when treating a trauma patient, some decisions need to be made rapidly, without the benefit of an in-depth discussion with all people involved.

After the cutover period, the smart change leader takes time to "mend fences." This could be writing notes, discussing issues, going to lunch, arranging a social get-together, etc. In the win-win philosophy this is relationship building and is needed to support future effort.

Conclusion

This chapter focused on sound approaches for managing some of the end stage aspects of the health informatics project. Organizations run on relationships and the smart informatics leader cements these relationships by showing appreciation to people for their past efforts and support and by building for the future. While many people say they do these end stage activities, they often treat them as anticlimactic or pro-forma. Our suggestions are offered to help change leaders be more effective in the long term.

Questions

1. Why is "just in time" training so important for a successful health informatics implementation?
2. What are some specific ways that organizations might celebrate a new health informatics system? Why is the celebration process so important?
3. What are some ways to avoid finger pointing when problems arise at cutover time?

4. Suppose you had the challenge of training physicians, nurses, and hospital administrative staff in the use of a new system. Would you use different training approaches for these three groups? How would they differ?
5. What are several end-stage communication strategies and processes that might work well in your organization?

Reference

1.   Naisbitt, John. *Megatrends: Ten New Directions Transforming Our Lives.* New York: Warner Books, 1982.

15
Evaluating Project Success

As the social action programs of the 1960s and 1970s developed and expanded, social scientists developed evaluation techniques and methodologies to help assess the outcomes of these programs. Evaluation became a requirement for many social programs and a key requirement of federally funded applied research efforts. Many of the social action programs of the time were in the health care field, and many if not all of the major health care organizations participated in these programs with their required evaluation components. However, only a minority of these health care organizations elected to apply their acquired evaluation skills to their internal programs and efforts. The concept of evaluation has progressed to where it is a very sophisticated system and one that provides valuable information to the decision makers.

Today, evaluation research is used in the area of outcomes research, which has been discussed for many years by a few people in the health care field. It is only recently that medicine has begun to accept and actively use outcomes research, which can be applied to the evaluation of the practice of medicine, with the intent that more-informed decisions can be made by both the physician and the patient.

There are many books and articles written on the principles and methods of evaluation. This chapter is a brief overview of evaluation and its role in health informatics information system implementation.

Critical Evaluation Issues

In evaluating health care informatics implementations, there are three critical questions, which are symbolically illustrated in Figure 15.1 using an analogy of darts and targets. In the top portion, which of the three targets is the correct one for our organization—the left, the right, or the center? In the middle portion, how close do we come to hitting the bull's-eye on the target that has been selected? In the

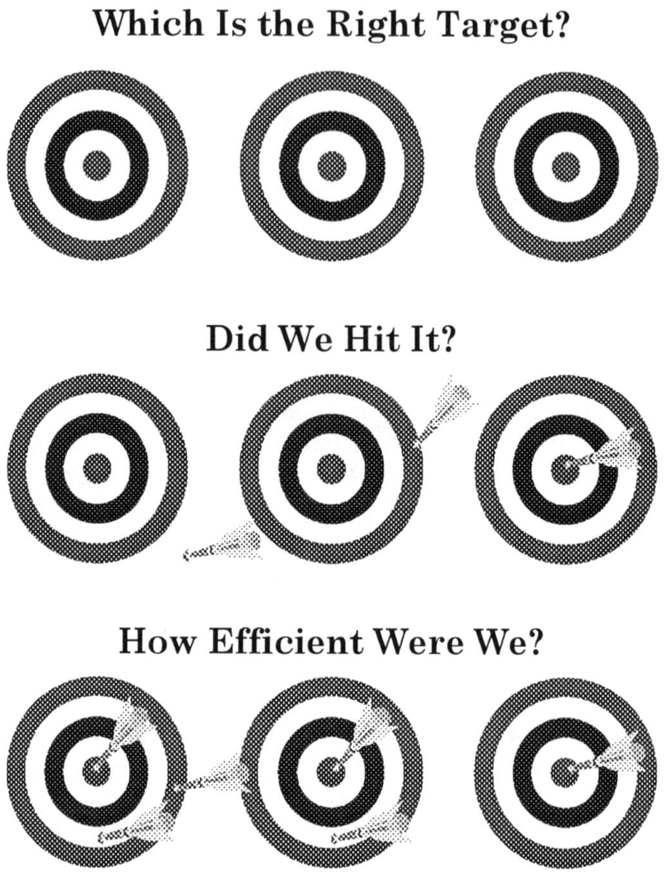

Which Is the Right Target?

Did We Hit It?

How Efficient Were We?

Figure 15.1. Three critical evaluation issues.

bottom portion, how many darts, i.e., resources, does it take us to hit whatever has been defined as acceptably close to the bull's-eye? Keeping these three concepts separate is critical in thinking about evaluation. If these three are confounded in the evaluation process, the interpretation of any outcomes is of questionable value.

What Does Evaluation Really Mean?

Basically, evaluation and evaluation research are concerned with determining out how well something works or how well something has been accomplished. That "something" could be an information system, a department within a hospital, a particular service, etc. Evaluation represents the application of social science research methods to discover information of importance about the program, practice, or department. This information can then be translated into future action.

Evaluation is undertaken to respond to areas of concern, such as

+ analysis of an existing situation and development of a projected ideal,
+ justification of a current or proposed activity, and
+ analysis of the quality of an activity or operation.

One classic definition of evaluation is "the process of ascertaining the decision areas of concern, selecting appropriate information, and collecting and analyzing information in order to report summary data useful to decision makers in selecting among alternatives."[1]

This definition of evaluation is based on the following assumptions:

+ Evaluation is an information-gathering process.
+ The information collected will be used mainly to make decisions about alternative courses of action. Therefore, the collection and analysis procedures must be appropriate to the needs of the decision makers.
+ Evaluation information should be carefully presented to the decision makers in a useful form with great care taken to avoid confusing or misleading them.
+ Different kinds of decisions will often require different kinds of evaluation procedures.[1]

Since health care organizations are in the business of trying to improve the human condition through a variety of organizational efforts, they are always making changes in services, departments, information systems, and so forth. An evaluation of those efforts is important to prove the value of the program or service. An evaluation of a health informatics system is needed not only to prove its value, but to determine if the system is doing what was intended originally.

The question in the health informatics area is how well do the programs implemented succeed in achieving the goals for which they were established? While this seems like a logical question, not everyone either wants to take the time or is interested in the answers. People may say, "The current system is working, and the technology is not available to do what they want." "We cannot ask the clinicians because we do not have the money for a new system anyway." "Leave well enough alone." Thus, those responsible for information systems sometimes do not see the need to evaluate since they have either little desire or little perceived ability to change things.

However, there comes a point for most information system leaders when it is important to ask these questions:

* "How are we doing in general?"
* "Are we accomplishing what we set out to do?"
* "Are we meeting our end users' needs?"
* "Are we keeping current technically?"

A crisis may precipitate this inquiry—shortage of funds, competing needs, obvious failures, etc. The senior leaders may want to know if they are getting their money's worth. In the case of a new information technology system, there is often a concern with learning whether the new system represents a good approach or are any changes needed. Sometimes the information systems staff members want to learn how to improve their effectiveness.

When there is serious interest in determining how well the information system is working, the evaluation can proceed by several routes. The processes are often somewhat foreign to those schooled primarily in the "hard sciences" who are used to working with variables that are more precisely measurable in physical terms.

> One way is through an impressionistic inquiry: an individual, a team, or a committee can go in and ask questions. Proceeding much as a good journalist does, the investigators talk to the program director, staff members, and recipients of service (students, clients, patients). They sit in on sessions, attend meetings, look at reports, and usually in a few weeks or months come up with a report. Much useful information can be ferreted out in this way, but the procedure has obvious limitations. It relies heavily on what people are willing to tell, and if the investigators are people from outside or upstairs—who can punish the program for inadequacies or departures from 'the book'— the flow of information is likely to be far from candid. The journalistic inquiry depends, too, on the skill and insight of the investigators, and on their objectivity. If they are rushed, bland, or biased, their assessments can be wide of the mark. Perhaps the most significant disadvantage is the focus on the here and now. Whatever the merit of its findings, the investigation usually can tell little about *outcomes* of the program—what effect it has in helping

participants achieve the goals for which the program was undertaken.

Another assessment technique is to administer question-naires or interviews that ask people's opinions about the program. Superficially, this appears more scientific and objective than the first type of investigation, and it does prevent the more patent intrusion of observers' biases. On the plus side, it also yields clues about program strengths and weaknesses. But again, as a method of evaluation, it is limited by what people divulge and by their immediate time perspective.[2]

Information systems generally aim to provide people access to information that they need as accurately and rapidly as possible. Evaluation is the process needed to determine if the goals and expectations of the system were actually achieved.

The Link to Expectations

When beginning an informatics evaluation process, it is important (1) to have a baseline assessment of the current system and (2) to link the evaluation to the comparison of outcomes to expectations. Before any organization decides to implement a new health information system there are usually specific organizational expecta-tions and goals for the new system. An evaluation will help organizations determine if the new health informatics system matches those initial systems expectations.

An evaluation process usually has three components: (1) an information-gathering section, (2) an assessment of the information gathered, and (3) a decision or future action component. To better enable the organization to make future decisions, the evaluation process should be started at the very beginning of the development or acquisition process for a new health information system.

Baseline Analysis

To determine the real impact of any new system, it is important to measure where the organization is before the development or acquisition process begins. It is necessary to measure the state of the systems and the information flows before any action is taken. While the need for baseline information is important, practical reasons may prevent the baseline data from being collected. For example, the top managers may feel that immediate action is needed and that they cannot wait for a systematic evaluation. Another reason might be that the organization does not have the resources—money or people—to complete an evaluation of the current system.

One of the major benefits of a baseline evaluation is that it can help the change leader and the senior leaders thoroughly understand the current system and determine if the direction they are considering will meet the needs of the organization and its people. Another benefit is that the baseline information may be helpful after implementation to prevent spurious comparisons of the new system to the old one. This can come in handy if people start reminiscing about the "good old days" and how wonderful things were before this terrible new system was installed.

When evaluation is not considered until the new system is being installed or completed, the opportunity for an accurate baseline evaluation is lost. Those charged with post-system evaluation must rely on retrospective reports, with all the risks of memory distortions, or on whatever documentary evidence happened to exist for other reasons at the time the decision to implement the new system was made. Such evidence is usually inadequate. Sometimes baseline measurements are incomplete simply because of lack of experience and foresight about what data might be needed later.

System Expectations

Before an organization makes a commitment to changing an information system or to installing a system where one does exist, there are usually many hours of discussion and a clarification about the goals and expectations for the system. Organizational vision and needs are discussed, probable system costs are examined, and many organizational levels and people are consulted before final approval occurs.

In Chapter 7, we discussed the issue of setting realistic systems performance expectations. To complete an effective evaluation of the new information system and the implementation process, it is essential that these realistic system expectations be clarified and used in the evaluation process as a measure of success or failure. The system expectations should be known to all involved in the system design and selection process. The expectations need to be written in simple declarative "capable of" statements, which are in turn used to develop evaluation questions and the evaluation methodology.

Evaluating the Implementation

The process of the system implementation is very important. Was the process smooth and without stress? Did the physicians and nurses actively participate and feel involved in the process? Did events happen as planned? What were the strengths and weaknesses of the manner in which the implementation occurred? These process-type issues are included in evaluating the actual implementation of a new health informatics system.

To evaluate the actions and events that occurred in the implementation process, an actual and first-hand account of what is being done is important, especially if the system being implemented is for the total, complex health organization. Very often the strategies listed originally differ from what happens in the "heat of battle." The person charged with the evaluation cannot assume that the plans and the actual implementation were as stated. There are a number of reasons for the possible discrepancy, including unclear perceptions or wishful thinking on the part of the staff and unrecognized conflict between people or groups. Evaluation is another reason why a dynamic planning and control process as discussed in Chapter 7 is so important. In addition to the direct planning benefits, such a process also provides a historic project trail for evaluation purposes.

One of the most difficult tasks in completing an evaluation study is finding the best techniques for understanding a process and the effects it has on people and systems and for estimating the degree to which observed phenomena approach the objectives of the program. This process is made easier by clear definitions of the goals and objectives. A practical problem of measurement in many studies is that of obtaining usable information. The application of evaluation techniques to the topic of an implementation process is usually costly and time-consuming, but important in order to redirect future efforts.

Evaluating the Quality of the System

After years of work, the health informatics system is implemented. Does the system do what it was originally designed to do? Is the system providing the type of information needed? What are the strengths and weaknesses of the system itself? The types of information that must be gathered in the evaluation of the system focuses on the system and how well it performs and meets expectations.

The same techniques and issues apply to the evaluation of the actual health informatics system as apply to the evaluation of the implementation process. The collecting, analysis, and presentation of data and information about the effectiveness of the new information technology-based system is important to determine if modifications are needed—in the system or in the redesign of the current process/information flow.

What Do We Do with the Information?

The underlying belief in evaluation efforts is that the study of the data, information, and communication collected furnishes the basis for constant feedback and readjustment of activities within the complex organization. The emphasis today is on building what are known as "learning organizations." In earlier days, the concept was often referred to as "learning loops" or "feedback loops."

The evaluation of complex organizations requires the formulation of objectives and criteria of accomplishment on a much broader scale. It is generally agreed that successful evaluation studies cannot be performed retrospectively, but rather must be built into the programs at their inception for true learning to take place. A number of considerations are advanced for such a position.

- When present from the beginning, the evaluation is less threatening, both because it seems part of the total process and because people come to feel they have had a hand in planning the evaluation.
- When skilled evaluators are an integral part of the planning phase of the system implementation, they can often help to improve the quality of the objectives as their attention is focused on the measurability of achievements.
- Experienced evaluators may be able to contribute substantively to the planning process by drawing on both their experiences and their knowledge of established social science findings. They may be able to suggest methods of known effectiveness and point out known difficulties in both the current operations and the system under development.
- Evaluators who are present from the start can follow the entire system and implementation process through planning, pretesting, and full-scale operations, thereby gathering information and keeping records of actual happenings.

Some organizations have established process action evaluation teams that may be made up of nurses, ward clerks, other unit staff, etc. The role of this team is to observe the day-to-day operations of the implementation process and to maintain a diary on the use and behavior of the system after it has been fully implemented. There are many ways for organizations to gather data. However, the key is using the data that has been gathered to make positive, proactive changes in the way systems are implemented within the organization and in the way that systems are designed and selected in the future.

Once the information from the evaluation is gathered and analyzed, it must be interpreted and summarized. Sometimes the results of the evaluation are best communicated in small doses, allowing changes to be introduced gradually rather than abruptly. This approach reduces the resistance to any changes. If the people who did the evaluation remain as closely connected to the effort as possible and help the change leader and senior leaders interpret and implement the findings, the results of the evaluation are more likely to be adopted than if a report is dropped in the lap of the change manager with no provision made for explaining findings or helping implement action steps.

Conclusion

To evaluate means to assess value. Before the assessment can take place, the desired value must be understood. Evaluation criteria may include the following: "(1) To monitor a steady state so as to determine when a correction is necessary. (2) To identify alternatives in a problem (non-steady) situation and provide relevant information. (3) To weigh alternative courses of decision-making in terms of relative gains and losses. and (4) To determine corrective action and the error-risks involved in various approaches to change."[3]

To study the problem of changing human behavior through evaluation, it is necessary to use applied and practical components of evaluation methods, which can examine the topic at hand. The number of such components is limited, and the huge variety of behavior-change techniques utilized are variations on a few central themes. The heart of evaluation is listening to people and using their input to change the system in a meaningful way.

Questions

1. Many organizations implement information systems without collecting baseline data. Why is this a poor long-term strategy?
2. What are the most important reasons for evaluating a health informatics system?
3. What might be several strategies for evaluating the power relationships in the organization before and after the health informatics system has been implemented?
4. "A bunch of opinions aren't really data." How would you respond to this comment?

References

1.   Alkin, MC. Evaluation theory and development. *Evaluation Comment* 1969;2:2–7.
2.   Weiss, CH. *Evaluating Action Programs: Readings in Social Action and Education.* Boston: Allyn and Bacon, 1972.
3.   Suchman, EA. Action for what? A critique of evaluative research. In O'Toole, R, ed. *Organization Management and Tactics of Social Research.* Cambridge: Schenkman, 1970.

16
Managing the Altered Organization

Remember "After the Ball Is Over," the classic Jerome Kern song from *Show Boat*? Well, what do *we* do when the music stops? Eventually all of our "how to" implementation concerns will be over, and our new health informatics system will be operational. If the system is a significant one, the organization will be affected as shown in Figure 16.1. As the health informatics projects are successfully implemented within an organization, the organization itself is altered. This, in turn, means that successful management of this "altered" organization may require different attitudes, controls, procedures, policies, and so forth.

Anyone who has been present when e-mail has been implemented in an organization has seen an example of an organization being altered by technology. Communications patterns typically change for both better and worse. E-mail promotes speedy informal communications that are nonintrusive compared with the telephone or in-person visits. On the other hand, some people can use e-mail to hide, trying to avoid organizationally desirable or necessary in-person communications. Also, some people lose their sense of restraint and engage in negative e-mail behaviors such as "flaming" others. E-mail often attacks the traditional hierarchical communication patterns, informally "flattening" the actual function-ing of the organization. As these organizational behaviors change, so do the required managerial behaviors.

Our increased understanding of altered organizations reflects the trend pointed out in 1985 by Paul Strassmann.

> The usual approach to dealing with the effects of informa-tion technology is to first examine its supply side, which includes technology of computers, software, communica-tions, information services, applications, databases, print-ers, memory devices, and so forth. For the last twenty-five years we have been preoccupied with such supply-side issues. To venture a guess, probably over ninety-five of every hundred pages of text written about office automation

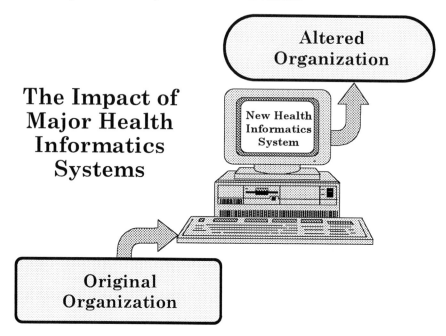

The Impact of Major Health Informatics Systems

Figure 16.1. The impact of health informatics implementations.

have dealt with these aspects. In the past, this amount of attention was appropriate because the technological capabilities were the key to getting anything accomplished. As a consequence, the audience of all this technical knowledge was concentrated among the two million technologists involved with the design, manufacture, and application of office automation devices. The actual users of computers could absorb only small doses of useful knowledge about computers from this literature.[1]

Shoshana Zuboff[2] also extensively studied information technology in the workplace. One of her conclusions is that the fully integrated workplace may not be a place at all, but "an arena though which information circulates." She says that intelligence is then applied to this "circulating" information and that from the intelligence process comes, "the quality, rather than the quantity, of effort [that] will be the source from which value is derived." She calls this the "informated" workplace and stresses how computers will change it. Zuboff's comments are especially interesting when we look at the knowledge networked organizations that were envisioned under the IAIMS (Integrated Academic/Advanced Information Management

Systems) program of the National Library of Medicine. The IAIMS vision stressed a fully integrated workplace with an interconnection of the education, patient care, and research functions of the health care setting. In the integrated information management world, each person would have a "front-end" access point to the knowledge network and that front-end system would be customized to the person's specific information needs, having the look and feel that is most useful and comfortable. In the IAIMS model, those who need information would be able to acquire it from wherever it was located. They could repackage the information as needed and could also apply intelligence to it to make appropriate decisions, whether for clinical care, education, research, or strategic direction.

Today, Davenport says, "information managers must begin by thinking about how people use information, not how people use machines."3 Davenport, arguing that the primary reason for information technology failure is that few companies have considered how people actually use information, developed the following ten item list entitled, "The Information Facts of Life."

1. Most of the information in organizations—and most of the information people really care about—isn't on computers.
2. Managers prefer to get information from people rather than computers; people add value to raw information by interpreting it and adding context.
3. The more complex and detailed an information management approach, the less likely it is to change anyone's behavior.
4. All information doesn't have to be common; an element of flexibility and disorder is desirable.
5. The more a company knows and cares about its core business area, the less likely employees will be to agree on a common definition of it.
6. If information is power and money, people won't want to share it easily.
7. The willingness of individuals to use a specified information format is directly proportional to how much they have participated in defining it or trust others who did.
8. To make the most of electronic communications, employees must first learn to communicate face-to-face.
9. Since people are important sources and integrators of information, any maps or models of information should include people.

10. There is no such thing as information overload; if information is really useful, our appetite for it is insatiable.[3]

Davenport's ten points—as well as the rest of his article—stress one of the major points of this book. Namely, the majority of us need to abandon our fixation with the hardware and software technologies and look at the people and the organizations and the information needs of both. We will always need those who focus on hardware and software development; however, with modern technologies, most of our organizations will require fewer, not more, of these narrow specialists.

In less than ten years, we have progressed from Strassmann to Zuboff to Davenport in terms of appreciating the role of information in organizations. We believe that this trend to understand and appreciate the people and their information needs will continue to grow as more people realize that taking control of the people and organizational issues is more important than any of the technologies that are purchased. Organizations have collectively spent billions of dollars on the technology, which is only one aspect of the information-people-machine interface (see Figure 1.2). In the future, we will have fully integrated information systems in health care organizations, but these systems will only come about with sound management of the people and organizational issues.

The Post-Implementation Organization

The change leaders may be so excited about the changes that the new technology will bring that they sometimes forget an important factor. For those who have not lived with the planning and development of the new system on a day-to-day basis, there will appear to be almost *instant* workplace changes. This is similar to the actor or actress who after 15 years of professional acting becomes an "overnight success." The public is completely unaware of the pain and trauma that the person experienced over the previous 15 years. All they see is the here and now—the big change.

The completion of the installation of an integrated information technology system will change the workplace. The changes may be in the way medicine is practiced; in the way patients are billed; in the way tests are scheduled; in the way test results are reported and received; or in the way physicians, nurses, or pharmacists are educated. We also know that there will be change-resistive behaviors and that it is important for the change management leader to develop effective strategies to help the organization and its staff adapt.

Once the system is fully integrated, you will learn how change-resistant some people's work behaviors are within the organization. No matter how "bad" the old system was or how much they complained about the old system, it was the system that they knew. They knew the system's quirks and foibles and how to make it work. The new system is unknown! People must change their day-to-day activities. Old habits must be changed to accommodate the new system and the new methods just when people were getting used to the old system.

After reviewing the literature for information about the post-implementation organization, our informal estimate is that over 95 percent of the materials we reviewed dealt with "getting there," i.e., the journey. We found very little information available on what to do or how to behave after arrival at the transformed state. Extending the travel analogy, it is as if we planned a trip and made arrangements only for the trip itself. However, we have no reservations or other arrangements for our stay at the destination. We don't even know what to pack. Most travelers realize the importance of information about the destination and doing some appropriate planning. Therefore, they read travel books or talk to travel agents or experienced travelers, seeking information and advice. We in the health informatics area need to put more energy and resources into analyzing the post-implementation organization so that we can do a better job of helping people understand what they will experience when they "arrive." At this stage of evolution in health informatics systems , the new types of organizations have not yet been identified, defined, and categorized. This is a major challenge for all of us who study health informatics.

Some Post-Implementation Issues

The post-implementation environment will face a variety of different issues, some internal and some external. Internally, we project that *organizational complaints* will be an issue in the early phases of the new organization. This will be followed by two issues: the recognition of and paying attention to the *power shifts* that will occur within the organization and the *access to information* phase. Externally, two major issues will face the post-implementation organization: the first is *alliances,* and the second is the recognition of the potential benefits to the organization's customers—patients, physicians, nurses, staff, community, and so forth.

Organizational Complaints

A new hospital was built to replace one that had been inadequate in various ways for some time. When the new hospital was opened, the patients were then transferred section by section. All the patients and visitors were impressed with the new facility. Not only was the physical plant outstanding, the hospital had some of the latest and most sophisticated technologies available. Moreover, tremendous effort had gone into ensuring that these new systems would be patient oriented. To our surprise, we learned that the hospital was facing a problem, the majority of the staff liked the old hospital and the old way of doing things better. This staff had to address not only the issues of a new workplace and all the changes that the new building brought, but also the new information-based technologies that compounded the problem. These two major changes seemed to be too much change for a staff that was accustomed to a very old physical plant and a lower level of technology. While a lot of planning had been done relative to the patients, not enough planning had been done relative to obtaining staff ownership in the new processes.

While complaining is a natural part of human behavior, change leaders need to look at the type of complaints and take appropriate action. For example, the new hospital building coupled with stress over new technology changes caused very basic or core complaints from the hospital staff. These complaints need to be taken seriously and addressed through organizational development strategies. Examples of organizational development strategies that might be used in this circumstance are having the staff talk about their feelings in one-on-one sessions with trained organizational development specialists, sponsoring discussion or focus groups, selecting several of the informal opinion leaders who like the new environment to talk with others or to help explore the issues with their peers, and sponsoring ways to acknowledge the new changes through celebrations. These types of strategies have two major benefits. First, the organization gathers excellent information that can assist it with determining potential interactions with its staff. Second, just as in the Hawthorne studies in the 1930s, when we pay attention to people and their practices, showing that we care, the people tend to respond in positive ways almost independently of the technical content of our interactions.[4]

The health informatics change leader cannot assume that the complaints will come from only lower-level staff. Some of those who will be the most reluctant to change will be the higher-level staff. In the case above, the major complaints were from physicians and nurses. The nurses aides and ward clerks liked the new system because they knew what they went through in the old system. Therefore, they took the time to learn and understand the capabilities of the new system, unlike the physicians and nurses who felt that they did not want to change the way they interacted with their patients. The complaints seemingly were about the details of the technology; however, the true complaint of the physicians and nurses was not wanting to undergo a second order change.

The health informatics change leader must (1) be aware of these human quirks of others (not any of us, of course) and (2) begin early to develop strategies to effectively manage workplace complaints that will occur. Most of the ways to address these issues involve *listening* to the complainers, not merely telling them that they will soon "get used to" the new system. Change leaders must be aware that it is part of our basic human need to "grumble" about things. It is more comfortable for people to talk to one another about problems and less comfortable to talk about the good things that are happening with the system.

Power Shifts

The post-implementation organization will be more people-sensitive and less bureaucratic. The organizations will be more cooperative and less hierarchical. Information technology will allow this organizational and behavioral set to emerge. This will be the true "high-tech and high-touch" phenomenon that has been discussed for a number of years. In turn, however, this causes some shifts in organizational power.

According to Rosabeth Moss Kanter,[5] bureaucracy tends to be position-centered while a post-entrepreneurial organization tends to be more person-centered with authority deriving from expertise or from relationships. She goes on to say that bureaucratic management is repetition-oriented, seeking efficiency through doing the same thing over and over. Post-entrepreneurial management is creation-oriented, seeking innovation as well as efficiency.

Many health care environments currently follow a "stove-pipe" management structure. Namely, people of like disciplines report to someone in their discipline, regardless of the area in which they actually work. For example, under this model, nurses in the emergency medicine department report to the director of nursing rather than to the director of emergency medicine. The same is true for the radiology technicians or laboratory technicians who work in the emergency medicine department. The stove-pipe model causes a complex bureaucracy to develop, with formal or informal protocols of who talks to whom. In the post-implementation organization everyone (within confidentiality restrictions) will have the capability to access the needed information for patient care and it will not matter where the person reports. To follow the example of the emergency medicine department, there could be a coordinator of emergency medicine services, thus eliminating much of the bureaucracy. As this type of definite power shift occurs, some of the people who were the directors in the stove-pipe system will fear that their power is diminishing, causing them anxiety.

Another type of power shift will occur within the professional disciplines. Prior to fully integrated information systems, many professionals gained and maintained power through their professional knowledge. For example, patients admitted to a hospital are often prescribed a number of drugs. The interaction of the various drugs with each other, with food, and on the various tests that are performed is important information for the clinicians to know. In the past, hospital pharmacists were the prime resource for this information. In a first order change, several excellent information packages were created that offered all the information needed. These packages were available to the hospital pharmacists to help support their giving information to the physicians and nurses. In a fully integrated information system, these drug information packages will be available directly to the physicians and the nurses. The pharmacists need only be consulted for those special areas that are not included in the drug information portion of the system. This will cause a major power shift and role change for the hospital-based pharmacists. While most of them will welcome and accept these changes, some will feel that they no longer have the proper status within the health care team and will resent their "diminished" power role within the total organization.

Access to Information

When organizations are fully integrated electronically, everyone with an appropriate need will have access to the knowledge-based distributed information world, which will significantly change our health care organizations. The change will start with the refocusing of why the information is needed. Just as patient-centered data bases became important in the past, human-centered information management will be the primary focus of all the information technology systems in the future. All of Davenport's information facts of life will be considered and incorporated into the system.

The key word for the future will be *customized*. Products and services will be designed to allow customization to meet the specific information needs of the individual, whether a clinician or a patient-customer. The customization of the products will occur at the users' end. The conflicts between access to information and confidentiality will be resolved. The end users will all access the same data bases. There will be personal filters and information maps to facilitate easy and effective use. There will also be sophisticated information guides that replicate some of the roles of librarians. The information managers in the future will be comfortable living in the world of ambiguity and will be flexible in providing information to the users of the health informatics system.

Once the clinicians and other users of the health care system discover that the information system conforms to their needs and goals rather than forcing them to conform to the needs and goals of the system, they will feel very positive about the integrated system. The users of the health informatics information systems finally come to see the power of these systems. Clinicians are realizing that it is more and more difficult to keep up with the changes in health care. Once the systems are clinician-cordial, the systems will be viewed as a helpful tool and not as an obstacle to high-quality health care. Clinicians will readily use the systems and wonder how they ever functioned without them.

Alliances

Regardless of the type and extent of health care reform, it is apparent to even the most casual observer that health care systems cannot continue to operate in the future as they have in the past. In the United States, the current health care model has been illness and specialist dominated. As the emphasis continues to move more toward primary care and a wellness model, health care organizations of all types will need to look at forming alliances. These alliances will allow the various organizations or groups to organize themselves in a variety of ways to meet the new-world health care order and have a high focus on quality care at a cost-efficient price. Alliances are coalitions that will allow organizations to meet the challenges of the new health care environment.

These new alliances will be an opportunity to create synergy for the people involved within the various organizations and within the new system that is created. The synergy created will lead to the development of new products and services for the patients and customers of the new health system. Synergy allows the staff and the leaders to add value to their products and services by building connections and adding quality to the various services that are offered within the organization.

Health informatics information management systems will directly support the success of the alliance. The systems will provide the needed information to enable the alliances to make the appropriate business decisions and to determine which direction is best for the total system in the new world order. Organizations will not have to function in the future on intuitive information; they will have accurate information on which to base decisions.

Customer Relations Changes

Without patients, where would the health care system be? But in the past, patients were often not included in decisions about their diagnosis and treatment. Yes, treatment options were offered; however, patients typically followed their physicians' recommendations. Even though the physician might continue to give statistical-based responses, there was usually a moment when the patient would assume that the physician was offering advice and would accept that advice. Patients signed consent forms, even though they did not fully understand the potential impact of the medical procedures, because they thought it was required, and they needed treatment. Issues of radiation tests from the 1960s and 1970s have raised the need for consent forms that indicate that the patients really understand the scope of the procedures for their diagnoses and treatments. More than thirty years after some of the early experiments with radiation to treat cancer, people have raised the issue that their relatives did not know that the tests were experimental.

Technology will provide a major means to communicate with patients. The patients will be directly involved with their diagnosis and treatment. They will use outcomes research systems that are information technology based and that will enable the patients to see the potential outcomes of the various treatment options. Patients will make their decisions based on their personal needs and not the general projected assumptions of their needs by the health care providers. The use of this patient-friendly information technology will assist not only in the treatment of patients, but also where appropriate in assisting patients with changing their lifestyles.

The health informatics systems will allow for the triumph of the individual patient. The technology will empower the health care professional not only to access readily the information that they need but to convey that information directly to the patient, no matter where he or she is located. The world will be tethered with global "tele" systems—telecommunications, televisions, telephones, etc.

The health informatics systems will emphasize the need to increase the amount and quality of communications with the patients and other customers of the health care system. Health care providers will have to increase their active listening skills. They were trained to think in the terms of their own discipline language and they find it much easier to talk to those with similar training. Health care providers, especially physicians, are often not as comfortable communicating with patients. Technology now provides a nonthreatening medium to facilitate communication between physician and patient. For example, if both are looking at an interactive system with researched information—presented in an understandable format—they can communicate with each other by talking about what they are seeing presented by the technology.

People and Practices

The fully automated health system workplace will be very different than the one we know today. In many instances, instead of the patients being transported from place to place within the hospital, the health care team will come to the patient. Computer-based technology will enable this shift to a patient-centered environment.

The new health care environment will require more speed. While clinicians are taught to make rapid decisions, some decision makers and support staff do not follow the "rapid decision" model. In some health care bureaucracies, decisions seem to take forever. When the organization's strategic direction is known and information that is needed for decision making is really available, then it will be easier to make decisions rapidly. In some organizations today, accurate information is not readily available; thus, they rely on "crystal ball" decisions. Lacking a sound vision or necessary information, managers often procrastinate on decisions, wanting to avoid mistakes. In some of these organizations, there is a tremendous amount of staff time directed to collecting needed information after the fact and for a specific purpose.

There will be more employee problem-solving teams to focus on identifying and eliminating any time wasters that get in the way of treating the patients. The continuous quality improvement (CQI) efforts will be integrated into the day-to-day operation of the health care system and thus will be not a program but an accepted way of life. As indicated in Chapter 8, some of the basic theories of sociology and psychology form the core of these CQI programs. Some people and organizations have already incorporated the social-psychology strategies into their day-to-day operating patterns. This will be true for the majority of health care enterprises in the future.

The information technology people will need to design and implement systems within this environment. They will need to follow a rapid prototype development model instead of the slower strategies and models that they have followed in the past. While the people trained in the information technology area may always be in love with the large mainframe computers and may always long for the "good old days," they need to move out of their shells and determine how the people or the organization will use the information they say they need. Some organizations may also follow the model of introducing the changes through a "research" unit, which will first design or adopt the information management strategies and technology needed. Then the technology will be gradually introduced into the total organization.

There will be fewer people within the health care environment and those that are available will need to complete more complex tasks. Technology will support future staff more and more. Some of the projections about the future show that people will not need to be located in one central site because they can function by telecommuting. These projections are not the same for the health care environment. Health care is a hands-on high touch world, and the clinical staff will usually need to be where the patients are. But in the future, doctors' hours will not be the 9 to 5 model. Physicians will be readily available during evening and weekend hours. Technology will help the physicians-patients-health settings to stay in close contact with each other. In the future doctors or nurse practitioners will even be making house calls; instead of having a black bag with a horse and buggy, they will have a high speed car with computers. Another future alternative is tele-medicine. Through the use of technology, a physician may be at a remote location and "see" the patient.

The future environment will leave the staff in a permanent hyperactive condition. In order to cope, the staff must be empowered to initiate and take appropriate action without involving a vast bureaucracy within the health environment. The people who live and work in this environment will feel the exhilaration of living on the cutting edge of the changes in health care and the application of the many new technologies that will be introduced into the health environment.

As we look into our crystal ball we see the majority of professional and support staff using technology to accomplish the majority of their tasks and responsibilities. We see the need for highly trained and committed people who are knowledgeable about the health system enterprise in which they work and are empowered to make the appropriate decisions as rapidly as possible. We see the need for the overall organizational behavioral culture to be the "high-touch and high-tech" model, with both reinforcing each other in a synergistic manner.

Leadership and Management

If our crystal ball assumptions are on target, we cannot continue to manage in the future as we have in the past. The post-implementation leaders must have the capability to develop trust and respect with their staff. The trust will come because the leaders not only have built a record of success, but also have developed enlightened people strategies. In the new environment, the leaders will trust and respect their subordinates, and in turn there will be a higher level of employee commitment. Trust will empower people and hold them accountable. Many times health care leaders and managers have relied on management behaviors that were used in the time of the heavily routinized work in very structured settings. These styles are usually high task and low interpersonal and come across as "whip crackers," as discussed in Chapter 10. This high task-low interpersonal approach is true for the traditional methods of educating our physicians as well as for managing in the inpatient and ambulatory care settings of the health system. However, these styles will not work in a fully integrated information environment. The values of trust and respect will dominate, and unfortunately, many of the managers of today will be unable to make the transition to the future.

We project that there will be fewer managers in the fully integrated information organization and that the future successful managerial styles will entail the high-interpersonal approach and could include either the high- or low-task approach, depending on the particular situation.

Integrated information management systems will facilitate the change in the role of management and leadership in the future. Probably the group that will be the most threatened in the future will be the middle managers. Health care institutions are notorious for having a high number of middle managers. An electronic-mail message contained the following statement. "On an average day in 1968, U.S. hospitals employed 435,100 managers and clerks to assist in the care of 1,378,000 inpatients. By 1990, the average daily number of patients had fallen to 853,000; the number of administrators and clerks had risen to 1,221,600." [6] It is our assumption that the majority of the people in the expanded group are middle managers, many of whom are technically competent but not well trained in management skills. While middle managers may be keeping the health care system moving today, with the advent of integrated information management systems and the use of more work teams, the number of middle managers will diminish.

There are so many health care issues that need attention. We do not have all the resources that we need; however, we seem to use many of our resources to either overmanage or manipulate workers in the health care system. The key to success for the leader and manager is the effective upgrading of the trust and respect for the hands-on workers within our organizations and the gradual extinction of the "whip cracker" school of management. This combination of changes in the organizational behavioral attitudes will benefit the customers of the health care enterprise, whether they are patients, students, staff, or ourselves. There is so much to do and not enough highly qualified people to do it; therefore, we need to practice intensively the value-based management discussed earlier. Organizations can create and reinforce this environment by clearly stating and then actively demonstrating what behaviors will be rewarded and what behaviors will be terminated. The resources will not be available in the future to cater to prima donnas, as we have done in the past in health care. We are all in the same boat—managers and staff—and we will sail or sink together.

The Learning Organization

The concept of organizational learning is not new. Almost twenty years ago, Chris Argyris was talking about double-loop learning.[7] Organizations are facing complex challenges from the scope of the changes in the health care system that are well beyond the realm of any individual to solve. Solving these problems will require many people to learn from each other and work together. In the double-loop organizations, individuals provide feedback to the people within the organization to help the individuals and organizations examine and change the underlying assumptions behind their actions.

Many researchers and academics have discussed organizational learning. We are not going to review that research; we merely want to stress that people and organizations can and do learn. As many of the day-to-day issues within the health care system are people related, organizational learning starts with core values management. This includes working with people in the organization in two major areas: (1) understanding the vision and direction of the organization, and (2) fully understanding the acceptable and unacceptable behaviors as well as the consequences of engaging in unacceptable behavior. Good parents know how to train and orient a child and when to express to a child that a certain behavior is unacceptable, e.g., for safety reasons. For the most part—at least until the teenage years—children listen and learn what is right and what is wrong. All too often, we do not practice this same type of socialization process, complete with consequences, within organizations. When managers see someone deliberately setting an "organizational fire" or slipping some "organizational poison" to another, the act is ignored to avoid conflict. Adults are educable; we *can* teach old dogs new tricks.

When we learn as individuals, we directly apply this learning to the organizational systems and processes, and then the organization learns. When our organization is troubled and plagued with dysfunctional behaviors, everyone in the organization must remember the words of that great American philosopher, Pogo, "We have met the enemy, and he is us!"

Conclusion

While we do not know exactly what the post-implementation fully integrated organization will be like, we do know that there will be major changes, both internally and externally, for these organizations. We expect these organizations will form more external alliances and that information will play a major role in the alliance-forming decision. Information systems will permit organizations to become learning organizations. The people and management practices of the future will need to change as the technology will permit the "high-tech and high-touch" concept to become a reality in the health care area. Professionals will be able to spend more time with their patients or customers and less time looking for information with which to make basic decisions. In the fully integrated information organization, we envision that professionals will be able to focus their energies on the meaningful portions of their professional activities more than they have ever been able to in the past. In fact, we envision that—like it or not—they will be forced to!

Questions

1. How would you envision an "informated" health care workplace operating in contrast to what exists today?

2. What kinds of power shifts do you see occurring in the fully integrated information organization?
3. What practical strategies do you think will help organizations improve their "learning" behaviors?
4. Describe what a typical nurse-leader's day might be like in the fully integrated information organization.
5. Do you agree that the number and role of middle managers will decrease in the fully integrated information organization? Why or why not?

References

1. Strassmann, PA. *Information Payoff: The Transformation of Work in the Electronic Age.* New York: Free Press, 1985.
2. Zuboff, S. *In the Age of the Smart Machine: The Future of Work and Power.* New York: Basic Books, 1988.
3. Davenport, TH. Saving IT's soul: Human-centered information management. *Harvard Business Review* 1994;72 (March-April):119–131.
4. Roethlisberger, FJ, Dickson, WJ. *Management and the Worker.* Cambridge: Harvard University Press, 1939.
5. Kanter, RM. *When Giants Learn to Dance: Mastering the Challenge of Strategy, Management, and Careers in the 1990s.* New York: Simon & Schuster, 1989.
6. McLinden, S, Cook, G. *Cook Report on Internet NREN.* 431 Greenway Avenue, Ewing, NJ 08618, (609) 882-2572, cook@path.net.
7. Argyris, C, Schon, D. *Organizational Learning: A Theory of Action Perspective.* Reading, MA: Addison-Wesley, 1978.

Section V
Future Issues

Introduction

This section represents our thoughts about health informatics in the future.

Chapter 17 begins with our visions about health informatics and systems. It also includes our predictions of some trends in both health informatics and information systems. The chapter ends with suggestions for organizational and personal preparation to meet the predicted trends.

17
Organizational and Personal Preparation for the Future

In listening to a retrospective audio tape about the professional life of the great sports announcer, Red Barber, it was interesting to hear him describe "announcing" the play-by-play description of an away baseball game in the early days of radio. Sports announcers in those days did not travel; therefore, Barber stayed in his team's hometown and learned about the game by reading the ticker tape. It was then his role to translate the information from the ticker tape into a "live" play-by-play commentary. In one particularly humorous anecdote, Barber describes what he had to do when the ticker tape stopped for a period of time when the game was at a particularly intense point.[1] While all this may seem ludicrous by modern standards, some of our antics and attempts at applying technology in health care will probably seem as ludicrous to future generations as trying to announce a baseball game without seeing it.

When we review any publication from ten, twenty, or fifty years ago, we sometimes laugh about the concern and consternation about what is standard operating procedure today. Young folks of today wonder what some of us did without videocassette recorders, let alone without televisions. They cannot imagine a world without some of the commonplace technologies that enhance our lives today.

Today, we face critical issues that will seem trivial if not laughable in future years. For example, we now worry about the confidentiality of the electronic patient record, even though we have not yet solved the confidentiality problem for the paper medical record. Computer-based records are increasingly necessary for quality patient care; however, confidentiality does not have to be compromised with the advent of new technology. The American Health Information Management Association, with more than 35,000 specialists in health-information management, is committed to the design and use of systems that protect patients' rights to the privacy and confidentiality of their health information. This group is working with the Computer-Based Patient Record Institute, the American Society for Testing and Materials, and the American Medical

Informatics Association Work Group on Electronic Data Interchange to design systems needed to ensure the privacy and confidentiality of computer-based patient records.

We are now in a transitional phase. Our vision of the future will become a reality—only the timing is still to be decided. As the great entertainer Jimmy Durante used to say, "You ain't seen nothing yet!"

A Vision of the Future

What can we realistically look forward to in the future? Based on our knowledge of technical and social trends, we present the following brief visions.

A Patient Vision

*   All medical-dental records will be in full electronic format, and each person will have a universal medical number.
*   The concept of the medical record will change from the disease-oriented record to a total personal health record containing information from wellness to illness. Our name for this record is PRIME (Personal Repository of Information of MEdicine).
*   The wellness approach to an individual's life will gradually predominate over the disease-model. Contained within each medical record will be a private "gene" map. Since the human genome will be fully mapped, it will be possible to create unique programs for both wellness and illness for an individual.
*   The electronic medical record will store visual information (e.g., radiographs, photographs, videos, etc.) as well as "printed" information.
*   Many of the testing procedures will be noninvasive. Surgical procedures will be greatly assisted by technology, especially lasers. A designer home-delivery model of health care will evolve from the complex of managed care, managed competition, resource management, and other health delivery systems.
*   Individuals will be regarded more as customers than patients, a natural evolution as the focus shifts to wellness. As customers, they will participate more actively in the decision process about their health behaviors and any treatments, if needed.
*   Access to computer-aided diagnostic databases will be through hand-held, voice activated devices that will offer guidance for possible problems, needed tests, etc. Computers will be at the point of interaction with the customers/patients and, with proper

authorization, will provide ready access to necessary information, including the patient's complete medical record.

+ Customer/patients will have on-demand access to sophisticated health education programs through narrowcasting technologies.
+ Scanners will be frequently used to diagnosis patient problems. The initial scanners will be called Star-Trek systems in honor of the television program that first introduced these systems more than forty years earlier.
+ Patients will be in control of their information and will participate with the health care provider in determining future directions.

A Research Vision

+ The use of animals in medical research will be very limited. The overwhelming majority of research tests will use simulation models.
+ Researchers will have mapped the entire human genome. Researchers will be able to assist the health care practitioners by designing special "patches" to fix gene problems or to develop designer drugs targeted to a specific problem.
+ While still very independent, researchers will spend most of their time researching the new and ever more complex disease entities. The AIDS pandemic will be over, but other pandemics will continue to occur with greater and greater speed given the "closeness" of the world and the extent of international travel and exchange programs.
+ Researchers will use ever more powerful computers to conduct their research and to maintain and manage the huge amounts of data their research will generate. Enhanced systems will predict if researchers are going to encounter problems or are on the verge of discovering new information.
+ Individual researchers will have extremely sophisticated, individual information algorithms to manage the wealth of information available to them electronically from anywhere in the world.
+ Major topic-specific research groups will be located throughout the world. To address the increasingly complex health issues, these groups will conduct large joint research projects. They will use extremely sophisticated telecommunications devices to communicate on a real-time basis for joint work.

An Education Vision

- The education of people for health-based professions will change drastically with heavy reliance on both technology and interpersonal learning methods.
- The changed health care environment will lead to a change in the ways in which students receive the clinical hands-on aspects of their education. Health care teaching professionals will have calculated the number and types of patients needed in order to teach students about the range of medical problems. Rather than students going on rounds or "working up" patients as admitted to a teaching hospital, students will be both placed with model practices and will also be entered into a patient's diagnosis and treatment at the appropriate time to give the patient the greatest amount of privacy.
- Virtual reality will be a major contributor to education in the future. For the health student (future physician, nurse, dentist, pharmacist, allied health, etc.) many of the educational modules will be built around virtual reality. ADAM & EVE is one example of the use of virtual reality in teaching human anatomy. By using the virtual ADAM & EVE model, students can take a trip through the human body and even do electronic "dissection." Another model called FIDO focuses on the anatomy of dogs. For those who remember the futuristic 1966 film, *Fantastic Voyage*, life will finally catch up with art in allowing "trips through the body."
- Health-based students will learn to practice medicine on life-size computer models, preprogrammed with a variety of both common and rare medical problems. The models communicate how they feel to the student nurses, physicians, pharmacists, etc. The models can develop adverse reactions to drugs, tests, etc. These models are more sophisticated extensions of the early computer-assisted instruction programs and the early voice-activated interactive videodisk programs. The models also have sophisticated interactive videodisk modules as database source for providing additional information to the students such as test results or x-rays.
- Continuing education for health care professionals will be greatly expanded. Professional reeducation will be mandatory. Every four years, health care professionals will have to reenter an educational enhancement program. Lifelong learning skills will be emphasized.

Knowledge Management

The Knowledge Network will be more fully developed, and there will be electronic (as well as human) mediators and "know-bots" that will help an individual navigate it. More sophisticated software will allow the end users of the electronic rivers of information to easily locate the information that they need for their patient care, research, or education needs. Knowledge management systems will allow the health workers to gain access to the vast array of information that exists regardless of its physical location.

Predicted Trends in Health Informatics

The visions discussed above were derived from the following predicted trends:

General

- The information systems in organizations will parallel the trends in their parent organizations; therefore, health informatics systems will not be oriented to just one health organization but will be interconnected to share information among alliance members.
- More of the mega-technologies such as cable systems and telecommunications will be integrated and will be available seamlessly wherever the information is needed—in the home, hospital, office, classroom, and so forth.
- All information technology systems will be more and more integrated.

Philosophy

- The knowledge and information contained in technology systems will be used as the prime filter for information system designs.
- More people will accept the importance of medical information and will either include it in their daily operational lives or alter their careers to work directly with medical informatics.
- Information will be viewed as a source of power in the reformed health care environment. Health care institutions will try to link more and more people and resources to their institutions through technology.

◆   In the new health care environment, the shift from acute-chronic care to preventive care will occur rapidly.

People

◆   People working in the health informatics areas will have more interdisciplinary viewpoints and will be more cooperative across disciplines.

◆   More high touch/human factors environments will be developed in the planning, design, implementation, and post-implementation aspects of new systems.

◆   End-user satisfaction will be a key measure of the quality and capability of the information system.

◆   The more that "high tech" systems enter the health care world, the more the demand will rise for the "high touch" aspects of health care delivery.

Products and Services

◆   Medical informatics will continue to provide more direct support for core services and products in health care, e.g., patient care, education, and research.

◆   Health care diagnosis and treatment will be available through tele-medicine or tele-health systems.

◆   Surgery will be performed in some cases without the "cutting" surgeon on site. As an aside, the rustic comedian Herb Shriner used to talk about coming from an Indiana town so small that there was no doctor. When someone needed surgery, they called Indianapolis with the patient's size and received back in the mail a pattern to lay over the patient. Then they just cut along the dotted lines. Now we have tele-surgery!

◆   More and more clinical databases will be available not only to health care professionals but also to the public.

Technology

◆   Control and access to information systems will be more widely distributed, yet unified.

◆   More sophisticated software technology and hardware technology will be available, but the systems will be much more user-cordial.

+ Bedside terminals and pocket computers will be used extensively in the treatment of the patient and will be wirelessly linked to host systems.
+ Scanners with Star Trek–level capabilities will become readily available.

Organizational Preparation to Meet These Trends

People, planning, leadership, and processes are the four most crucial elements for an organization as its prepares to meet these future trends.

People

+ The key to organizational success in the future will be the involvement of people in the health informatics area. All stakeholders will have an opportunity to participate in the assessment and design of future systems to ensure that their information needs are considered and addressed.
+ Technology will be used to encourage stakeholders to offer their opinions in a variety of formats—interviews, surveys, etc. The groupware survey technology will be more sophisticated. For example, people on all three shifts will be able to easily participate in any data-gathering process.
+ A key word for the future will be *customized*. Each person will be able to easily customize their interfaces with the systems they use in their daily work.

Planning

+ The use of rapid prototyping models will be the key to meeting the ever-changing organizational environment. Most organizational planning will use fast-track, yet people-intensive, methods. The fast-track planning methods start with a future vision process. The organization then positions itself strategically to meet their future vision.

Leadership

+ The leaders in organizations will assume that technology is the part of every job and will not have separate groups to process data or information. The information professional role will focus more on counseling and advising user areas on how to obtain maximum benefits from the available technologies.

♦ Those responsible for health informatics will be perceived as strategic leaders in their organizations, and their inputs will not be confined to the technology area. The leaders will focus more on the information needs of their wide range of "customers."

Processes

♦ In the future, organizations will have adopted the "learning organization" concepts that will link people more closely to the organizational vision. The involvement of people and their input and feedback will allow organizations to move more quickly—yet with less stress—as the people are actively involved in the process and take ownership in the new systems.

Personal Preparation to Meet These Trends

Hardware, software, philosophies, and the changes in health care are moving so rapidly that health informatics professionals must plan to educate themselves on a daily basis about the changes.

Let's look at practical strategies for the future. The following suggestions may seem a bit simplistic. However, the person who aggressively pursues these basic strategies will confront the information challenge proactively rather than reactively.[2]

1. **Be willing to change.** Abraham Lincoln said, "You cannot escape the responsibility of tomorrow by evading it today." In her excellent book, *Danger in the Comfort Zone*, Dr. Judith Bardwick discusses the bleak future facing those who feel they are *entitled* to continue working in the future as they have in the past. She is not talking about levels of effort. Many of the people she refers to work hard day-in, day-out. The tragedy is that their efforts are essentially worthless as they struggle to maintain a past that has been made irrelevant by change. According to Bardwick, "Only when there's a sense of danger do you get real energy and long term commitment to deal with the pain and anxiety of change."[3]

2. **Prepare yourself for the future.** Read at least one future-oriented article or book a week. Prepare yourself educationally—whether through formal courses or continuing education courses.

Know and understand the appropriate technologies and their trends.

Just as important, spend time with people to learn the technological trends in their areas. One of the keys to successful future informatics systems will be linking them much more closely to the specific technologies in the various areas of our total health care system.

3. **Define your mission**—the purpose for which your unit exists. Define what success strategies are best for you. Undoubtedly, you have heard Tom Peters quoted on this over and over. Well, if you don't believe Tom Peters, at least remember the words of Lewis Carroll:[4]

> "Cheshire Puss," Alice began rather timidly, "would you tell me, please, which way I ought to go from here?"
>
> "That depends a good deal on where you want to get to," said the Cat. "I don't much care where," said Alice.
>
> "Then it doesn't matter which way you go," said the Cat.
>
> "So long as I get somewhere," Alice added as an explanation.
>
> "Oh, you're sure to do that," said the Cat, "if you only walk long enough."

It doesn't make much difference which way you go if you don't have a specific end in sight.

4. **Set mission directed goals**—short, medium, and long range. First, you need to set some specific operational goals for yourself and then pursue them vigorously rather than letting yourself be caught up in fighting the fires.

What are specific goals? Specific goals tend to have the following characteristics:

- They are written.
- They are measurable.
- They are expressed in terms of results, not activities.
- They are realistic, challenging, yet attainable.
- They specify a period or date of accomplishment.

Once these goals are set, keep your eyes on them. Red Barber reminisced about Babe Hermann of the Brooklyn Dodgers. One day Babe was chasing a fly ball, when his cap flew off. Babe stopped and retrieved his cap, letting the fly ball fall safely for a

hit. Are there times when you fail to keep your eye on the ball and become distracted by the trivial?
5. ***Keep a list of your successes and failures.*** Every life has its victories and its defeats. Analyze both and learn from them. The key is maintaining perspective and not letting the defeats get you down. That is why it is so important to dwell on the plusses as well as the minuses.

Warren Bennis, a true leadership and management guru, stresses the importance of optimism. Bennis has told us that his organizational research shows that successful leaders—while they maintain a realistic view—look at a glass and see it as half full rather than half empty.

Conclusion

We are in the midst of concurrent technological information explosions. Megachange is occurring almost daily. Our desire for information continues to outstrip the ability of our systems to meet their needs. Users will always want more information than our technology of the moment will be capable of giving. However fast our technology evolves, users' needs will evolve even faster, requiring human expertise and intuition to guide information seekers along the fringes of the technology and into the inevitable gray areas between technologies.

Our goal is to maintain the balance between the high tech world that we live in and the high touch world that we all need.

Questions

1. What is your vision of how patient medical records will be handled in the future?
2. What are the physician information needs that your vision addresses?
3. What is your definition of the "knowledge network"?
4. Outline your personal preparation strategies for working in the increasingly complex health informatics area of the future.

References

1.   Brennaman, M. *Red Barber: From the Catbird Seat.* Cincinnati: WVXU, 1993.
2.   Lorenzi, NM. *High Wire Act.* Speech presented to South Central Chapter, Medical Library Association, Houston, Texas: October 25, 1992.
3.   Bardwick, JM. *Danger in the Comfort Zone.* New York: AMACOM, 1991.
4   Dodgson, CL [Carroll, L]. *Alice's Adventures in Wonderland.* New York: Delacorte Press, 1978.

Index

A

Abrahamson, James, 110
Ackoff, Russell, 88
ADAM & EVE, 298
Adaptive planning, 138
American Health Information
    Management Association, 295
American Medical Informatics
    Association, 296
American Society for Testing and
    Materials, 295
Anders, George, 39
Antennae, good manager's, 168–69
Argyris, Chris, 290

B

Bales, R.F., 152
Ball, Marion J., vii, ix
Bardwick, Judith, 303
Barnett, G. Octo, 224
Baseline data, 128
Belasco, James, 157
Benchmarking, 85
Bennett, George, 97
Bennis, Warren, 96, 304
Benson, H., 253
Blanchard, Kenneth, 194, 198
Blue Cross/Blue Shield, 43
Boyett, Joseph, 80

C

Capable of statements, 90
Carlisle, Arthur Elliott, 196
Carroll, Lewis, 303
Change

critical issues for, 78–79
first-order, 22
levels of, 22–27
making informatics enable, 115
megachange, 27
microchange, 27
middle-order, 23
proactive vs. reactive, 79
second-order, 23
testing organizational readiness
    for, 96–116
types of, 27–28
Change management
change theories, 155–57
definition of, 150
related to stress, 21
strategies, 157–60
Change theory, 150–52
theory of groups, 151
theory of logical types, 151
Changing information environment,
    35–38
Chief information officer
acid test, 114
and sabotage, 215
areas of responsibility, 113–14
education and training, 189
losing trust, 113
negative example, 3
role of, 60, 70–71, 106
Childs, W., 227
CIO, *see Chief information officer*
COBOL, 7
Comfort zone, 20
Communications
as middle manager role, 262
as political necessity, 176–77

as responsibility of CIO, 113
effects of e-mail, 277
end stage, 259–61
evaluation results, 275
in larger units, 65
in small units, 64
of priorities, 141
of values, 142
organizational vision, 219
technology diffusion, 216
through interdisciplinary focus
groups, 220
to end users, 95
to staff, 55
two-way, 177
with patients, 286
with project management tools,
136
within small group, 152
Communications among subunits,
55
Compleat manager, 168–69
Computer-Based Patient Record
Institute, 295
Conflict, types of (Lewin), 154–55
Conflicts between professionals,
228–31
Conn, Henry, 80
Consultant competency, 8
Continuous quality improvement,
27, 76, 80, 150, 287
Coping with system shortcomings,
263–64
fixable problems, 264
unfixable problems, 264
Corporate culture, see
Organizational culture
Covey, Stephen R., 247–52
CQI, see Continuous quality
improvement

D

Dalziel, Murray, 177
Davenport, T.H., 57, 279, 280, 284
David, Paul A., 36

Dearden, Robert, 218
Delphi approach, 131
Deming, W.E., 79
Dixon, Bradley, x, 112, 114
Double-loop learning, 290
Dowling, Alan, x, 215
Dreyhaupt, Ken, x
Drucker, Peter, 191, 210
Dun & Bradstreet, 88

E

End stage issues
breaking down barriers, 263
celebration, 261
communication, 259–61
coping with system
shortcomings, 263–64
desirable pattern, 257
mending fences, 264–65
traditional pattern, 256
training and support, 257–59
End users' needs, 95–96
Ernst and Young, x, 215
Evaluation
and system expectations, 272–73
assumptions underlying, 269
baseline analysis, 272
critical issues, 267–68
defined, 269
for outcomes research, 267
in health informatics area,
269–70
link to expectations, 271–73
of implementation process,
273–74
of system quality, 274
using the results, 274–75

F

Failures
definition of, 6
why they happen, 6–10
Features vs. benefits, 120
FIDO, 298
Field theory, 153–55

force fields, 154
Fisch, R., 150
Fischer, Thomas S., x, 139
Fisher, Roger, 250
Flexible systems, need for, 140–41
Force fields
    analysis examples, 156–57
Friedman, Meyer, 242
Future
    education vision, 298–99
    knowledge management, 299
    organizational preparation for,
        301–3
    patient vision, 296–97
    personal preparation for, 303–5
    research vision, 297–98

G

Gantt charts, 136
Gardner, John W., 62
Gateways, 121
General Motors, 43
Genome, 103, 296, 297
Glazer, Howard I., 245–47
Golembiewski, R.T., 23
Great idea, but . . ., 163
Greiner, Larry, 62, 63, 66, 68
Growth stages, see Organizational
    growth

H

Hall, Jay, 210
Hannah, Kathryn J., vii, ix
Harrison, Donald C., ix
Hawthorne studies, 282
Health care organizations
    competitive realities, 208–10
    current environmental forces,
        47–49
    differences from others, 38–46
    similarities to others, 46–47
Health care team, 228, 233–34
Hersey, P., 194, 198
High tech/high touch, 85, 259, 283,
    289, 291, 300, 305

Horak, Bernard, x, 128, 229

I

I really support this effort, but . . .,
    164
I support you fully, but . . ., 165
IAIMS, 13, 91–92, 223, 278
IBM, 120
IMIA Working Conference, 138, 215
Informated workplace, 278
Informatics principles, strategic,
    104
Information as change, 19
Information facts of life, 279–80
Information politics, 57–62
    anarchy, 59
    federalism, 61–62
    feudalism, 59–60
    monarchy, 60–61
    technocratic utopianism, 58–59
Information systems development
    modern approach, 119–20
    product development analogy,
        120–21
    traditional approach, 118–19
Initial productivity curve, 128–29
Installed base, 111
Involvement vs. commitment, 94
Issues, global vs. local, 84–88

J

Jay, Anthony, 185
Johns, Richard, 169

K

Kaiser Permanente, x, 139
Kanter, R.M., 96, 283
Katz, R.L., 75
Kenny, David A., 202
Kidder, Tracy, 117
Klekamp, Bob, 240
Klipper, M.Z., 253
Know-bots, 299
Knowledge network, 299
Krug, D., 196

L

Leadership commitment, need for, 94
Leadership continuum, 91
Leadership issues in medical informatics, 186–91
Leadership sources
  computer-based professionals, 187
  informatics educated/trained professionals, 188
  library-based professionals, 187–88
  technically educated/trained professionals, 188
  tinkerers, 188–89
Leadership styles
  and stages of growth, 193–202
  comparison of models, 199
  observed, 194–96
  OJRs, 194–96
  proactive vs. reactive, 196
  researched model, 194
  schmoozers, 194–96
  team builders, 194–96
  whip crackers, 194–96
Leadership success characteristics, 202–7
Leadership, organizational legitimization, 189–91
Learning organization, 290–91
Legacy systems, 7
Lewin, Kurt, 135, 153–54, 156, 157

M

Machiavelli, 166, 185
Management
  administration vs. leadership, 191
  competence and responsibilities, 191–93
  efficiency vs. effectiveness, 191
  specific roles, 192–93

Management levels, critical skills at, 75–78
Managerial checklist, 143–49
Managing expectations, 115, 129–30
Mantel, S.J., Jr., 117
Mary Smith scenario, 91–92, 95
Mazoue, James, 225
MBWA, 193
Meador, C.K., 42
Mending fences, 264–65
Meredith, J.R., 117
Mintzberg and Quinn model, 113
Mintzberg, Henry, 112, 192

N

Naisbitt, John, 70, 85, 259
National Health Service, 5
New systems, threats from, 19
Nurse culture, 225–26

O

Oakley, E., 196
Office of Technology Assessment, 214
Oracle, 110
Organizational culture, 54–57
  ideologies, 177–79
  measures, 55
  scale, 57
Organizational growth, stages of, 62–70
  and leadership styles, 196–98
Organizational issues
  traditional approach, 15–16
  why not given due, 13–15
Organizational skills, definition of, 12
Organizational structures, types of, 70–72
Organizational values, 55, 81–82
OSCAR, 4

P

Peel, Victor, x

People-ware strategies, 219–21
Perspective, maintaining sense of,
    174–75
Peters, Tom, 55, 303
Pharmacist culture, 226
Phillips, Karen, x
Physician culture, 224–25
Planning process
    adaptive plans, 138
    computerized tools, 135–36
    effective methods, 112–13
    example, 108–9
    health informatics issues,
        109–11
    organizational styles, 111–12
    people-ware track, 219–21
    plans as forecasts, 136–38
    politics in, 114–15
    resources needed, 135
    role of the CIO, 113–14
    who should be involved, 112
Pliskin, N., 55
Politics
    and power, 165–68
    avoiding isolation., 177
    examples of political problems,
        163–65
    in planning process, 114–15
    power people, 175–76
    rules of the game, 177–79
    silver bullets, using wisely,
        181–82
    twelve key strategies, 173–82
Porter, Michael, 112
Post implementation
    leadership and management,
        289–90
    people and practices, 287–89
Post-implementation organization,
    280–87
    access to information, 284–85
    alliances, 285–86
    customer relations changes,
        286–87

organizational complaints,
    282–83
power shifts, 283–84
Power
    derived power, 167
    formal and informal, 94
    interpersonal power, 166–67
    knowledge-expertise power, 167
    knowledge-information power,
        167
    positional power, 167
    referent power, 167
    sources of, 166–68
Primary group concept, 152
Problem-solving wheel, 192
Procter and Gamble, 68, 77, 129
Product development analogy,
    120–21
Productivity
    conditions for, 210–14
    people and, 210–14
Professional systems and culture,
    223–26
Professionals
    managing conflicts between,
        228–31
    system effects on, 226–28
Project
    desirable end stage pattern, 257
    six phases of, 117
    traditional end stage pattern,
        256
Project management
    add-on requests, 134–35
    budget, 9
    concurrent approach, 139
    critical concepts, 124
    key project values, 141–43
    laws of, 149
    managerial checklist, 143–49
    overall process, 122–24
    postmortems, 121
    scope, 9
    scope creep, 134–35
    shortcomings, 9–10

skills, 12
time, 9
tools, 9
total systems approach, 121–22

R

RCA, 120
Realistic estimates
    dangers of overselling, 132–33
    Delphi approach, 131–32
    need for database, 131
Realistic goals, setting, 120
Resistance to change
    cultural dimensions, 185–86
    important factors, 29
    intensity, 30–31
    types, 29
Riley Associates, 142, 143, 192
Rogers, E.M., 217
Rosen, Peter N., x
Rosenman, Ray, 242
Running a meeting, 152–53

S

Sabotage, 215–16
Schein, Edgar, 191
Schmidt, Warren, 90
Schoonover, Stephen, 177
Scott, Jim, 129
Seils, Andrea, x
Self-esteem, 20, 111, 129, 179, 180,
    205, 224, 238, 239, 252
Selye, Hans, 20
Sense of humor, 181
Sharks, swimming among, 169–73
Sheep and wolves, 127, 199–202,
    239
Sheppard, Blair, 185
Six silver bullets, 181–82
Sled dog model of team building,
    232–33
Slevin, Dennis, 168
Small group theories, 152–53
Sodana, Andrea, 97
Strassmann, Paul, 277, 280

Strategic informatics principles,
    104–7
    examples, 104–6
    key questions, 106–7
    relationship to overall planning,
        107–9
Stress
    and change, 96
    avoidance, 20
    relationship to change, 20–21
    vs. distress, 20
Stress management
    and feelings of control, 252
    and personality, 242–47
    and self-esteem, 238
    Glazer-StressControl life-style
        questionnaire, 245–47
    it's only a game, 237–39
    manufacturing trivial stresses,
        240–42
    positive vs. negative techniques,
        235
    possible negative effects of
        stress, 235–36
    relaxation response, 253–54
    role of exercise, 237–39
    sheep and wolves, 239
    standard tools, 247–52
    type A or type B personalities,
        242–47
    urgency vs. importance, 249–50
Successful system, definition of, 6
Swimming among the sharks,
    169–73
Symmetrix, 97
System improvement, stages of,
    21–22
System performance objectives,
    126–30

T

Tannenbaum, Robert, 90
Team building, 231–33
    sled dog model, 232–33

Teams, characteristics of effective, 231–32
Technical skills, definition of, 11
Technological innovation curve, 8
Technology strategies
  bleeding edge, 8
  leading edge, 8
  trailing edge, 8
Technology transfer
  diffusion concepts, 216–17
  stages of, 217–19
Theory of groups, 151
Theory of logical types, 151
This is really good, but . . ., 164
Time estimates, role of personality, 130–31
Top-down impositions, dealing with, 133–34
Total quality management, 80, 150, 219, 220
TQM, *see Total quality management*
Training
  fear of, 157
  for a CIO, 189
  just in time, 220
  medical, 224
  nursing, 225
  one-on-one, 159
  opportunities, 4
  residency, 224
  standardized programs, 61
  time required, 129
  tinkerers lack of, 189
  true cost of a PC, 149
  typical shortcomings, 15–16
  vs. change management, 138
Trends in health informatics, 299–301
  general, 299–300
  people, 300
  philosophy, 300
  products and services, 300–301
  technology, 301
Trojan horse, 215

U

Ury, William, 250

V

van Bemmel, Jan H., 186
Vendor competency, 8
Vendor misinformation, 110
Vision for change, creating, 88–92

W

Waterman, Robert, 55
Watzlawick, Paul, 22, 150, 151, 152, 217
Weakland, J.H., 150

Z

Zaccaro, Stephen J., 202
Zuboff, Shoshana, 278, 280